How To Treat And Control Asthma

314 Great Tips For Getting Quick Relief From Asthma

ADAM COLTON

Published by BizMove
www.bizmove.com

ISBN: 1978373899
ISBN- 978-1978373891

Table of Contents

1. Asthma Fact Sheet

What Is Asthma?

Asthma (AZ-ma) is a chronic (long-term) lung disease that inflames and narrows the airways. Asthma causes recurring periods of wheezing (a whistling sound when you breathe), chest tightness, shortness of breath, and coughing. The coughing often occurs at night or early in the morning.

Asthma affects people of all ages, but it most often starts during childhood. In the United States, more than 25 million people are known to have asthma. About 7 million of these people are children.

Overview

To understand asthma, it helps to know how the airways work. The airways are tubes that carry air into and out of your lungs. People who have asthma have inflamed airways. The inflammation makes the airways swollen and very sensitive. The airways tend to react strongly to certain inhaled substances.

When the airways react, the muscles around them tighten. This narrows the airways, causing less air to flow into the lungs. The swelling also can worsen, making the airways even narrower. Cells in the airways might make more mucus than usual. Mucus is a sticky, thick liquid that can further narrow the airways.

This chain reaction can result in asthma symptoms. Symptoms can happen each time the airways are inflamed.

Sometimes asthma symptoms are mild and go away on their own or after minimal treatment with asthma medicine. Other times, symptoms continue to get worse.

When symptoms get more intense and/or more symptoms occur, you're having an asthma attack. Asthma attacks also are called flareups or exacerbations (eg-zas-er-BA-shuns).

Treating symptoms when you first notice them is important. This will help prevent the symptoms from worsening and causing a severe asthma attack. Severe asthma attacks may require emergency care, and they can be fatal.

Outlook

Asthma has no cure. Even when you feel fine, you still have the disease and it can flare up at any time.

However, with today's knowledge and treatments, most people who have asthma are able to manage the disease. They have few, if any, symptoms. They can live normal, active lives and sleep through the night without interruption from asthma.

If you have asthma, you can take an active role in managing the disease. For successful, thorough, and ongoing treatment, build strong partnerships with your doctor and other health care providers.

What Causes Asthma?

The exact cause of asthma isn't known. Researchers think some genetic and environmental factors interact to cause asthma, most often early in life. These factors include:

- An inherited tendency to develop allergies, called atopy (AT-o-pe)
- Parents who have asthma
- Certain respiratory infections during childhood
- Contact with some airborne allergens or exposure to some viral infections in infancy or in early childhood when the immune system is developing

If asthma or atopy runs in your family, exposure to irritants (for example, tobacco smoke) may make your airways more reactive to substances in the air.

Some factors may be more likely to cause asthma in some people than in others. Researchers continue to explore what causes asthma.

The "Hygiene Hypothesis"

One theory researchers have for what causes asthma is the "hygiene hypothesis." They believe that our Western lifestyle—with its emphasis on hygiene and sanitation—has resulted in changes in our living conditions and an overall decline in infections in early childhood.

Many young children no longer have the same types of environmental exposures and infections as children did in the past. This affects the way that young children's immune systems develop during very early childhood, and it may increase their risk for atopy and asthma. This is especially true for children who have close family members with one or both of these conditions.

Who Is at Risk for Asthma?

Asthma affects people of all ages, but it most often starts during childhood. In the United States, more than 22 million people are known to have asthma. Nearly 6 million of these people are children.

Young children who often wheeze and have respiratory infections—as well as certain other risk factors—are at highest risk of developing asthma that continues beyond 6 years of age. The other risk factors include having allergies, eczema (an allergic skin condition), or parents who have asthma.

Among children, more boys have asthma than girls. But among adults, more women have the disease than men. It's not clear whether or how sex and sex hormones play a role in causing asthma.

Most, but not all, people who have asthma have allergies.

Some people develop asthma because of contact with certain chemical irritants or industrial dusts in the workplace. This type of asthma is called occupational asthma.

What Are the Signs and Symptoms of Asthma?

Common signs and symptoms of asthma include:

- Coughing. Coughing from asthma often is worse at night or early in the morning, making it hard to sleep.
- Wheezing. Wheezing is a whistling or squeaky sound that occurs when you breathe.

- Chest tightness. This may feel like something is squeezing or sitting on your chest.
- Shortness of breath. Some people who have asthma say they can't catch their breath or they feel out of breath. You may feel like you can't get air out of your lungs.

Not all people who have asthma have these symptoms. Likewise, having these symptoms doesn't always mean that you have asthma. The best way to diagnose asthma for certain is to use a <u>lung function test</u>, a medical history (including type and frequency of symptoms), and a physical exam.

The types of asthma symptoms you have, how often they occur, and how severe they are may vary over time. Sometimes your symptoms may just annoy you. Other times, they may be troublesome enough to limit your daily routine.

Severe symptoms can be fatal. It's important to treat symptoms when you first notice them so they don't become severe.

With proper treatment, most people who have asthma can expect to have few, if any, symptoms either during the day or at night.

What Causes Asthma Symptoms To Occur?

Many things can trigger or worsen asthma symptoms. Your doctor will help you find out which things (sometimes called triggers) may cause your asthma to flare up if you come in contact with them. Triggers may include:

- Allergens from dust, animal fur, cockroaches, mold, and pollens from trees, grasses, and flowers
- Irritants such as cigarette smoke, air pollution, chemicals or dust in the workplace, compounds in home décor products, and sprays (such as hairspray)
- Medicines such as aspirin or other nonsteroidal anti-inflammatory drugs and nonselective beta-blockers
- Sulfites in foods and drinks
- Viral upper respiratory infections, such as colds
- Physical activity, including exercise

Other health conditions can make asthma harder to manage. Examples of these conditions include a runny nose, sinus infections, reflux disease, psychological stress, and <u>sleep apnea</u>. These conditions need treatment as part of an overall asthma care plan.

Asthma is different for each person. Some of the triggers listed above may not affect you. Other triggers that do affect you may not be on the list. Talk with your doctor about the things that seem to make your asthma worse.

How Is Asthma Diagnosed?

Your primary care doctor will diagnose asthma based on your medical and family histories, a physical exam, and test results.

Your doctor also will figure out the severity of your asthma—that is, whether it's intermittent, mild, moderate, or severe. The level of severity will determine what treatment you'll start on.

You may need to see an asthma specialist if:

- You need special tests to help diagnose asthma
- You've had a life-threatening asthma attack
- You need more than one kind of medicine or higher doses of medicine to control your asthma, or if you have overall problems getting your asthma well controlled
- You're thinking about getting allergy treatments

Medical and Family Histories

Your doctor may ask about your family history of asthma and allergies. He or she also may ask whether you have asthma symptoms and when and how often they occur.

Let your doctor know whether your symptoms seem to happen only during certain times of the year or in certain places, or if they get worse at night.

Your doctor also may want to know what factors seem to trigger your symptoms or worsen them.

Your doctor may ask you about related health conditions that can interfere with asthma management. These conditions include a runny nose, sinus infections, reflux disease, psychological stress, and <u>sleep apnea</u>.

Physical Exam

Your doctor will listen to your breathing and look for signs of asthma or allergies. These signs include wheezing, a runny nose or swollen nasal passages, and allergic skin conditions (such as eczema).

Keep in mind that you can still have asthma even if you don't have these signs on the day that your doctor examines you.

Diagnostic Tests

Lung Function Test

Your doctor will use a test called <u>spirometry</u> (spi-ROM-eh-tre) to check how your lungs are working. This test measures how much air you can breathe in and out. It also measures how fast you can blow air out.

Your doctor also may give you medicine and then test you again to see whether the results have improved.

If the starting results are lower than normal and improve with the medicine, and if your medical history shows a pattern of asthma symptoms, your diagnosis will likely be asthma.

Other Tests

Your doctor may recommend other tests if he or she needs more information to make a diagnosis. Other tests may include:

- Allergy testing to find out which allergens affect you, if any.
- A test to measure how sensitive your airways are. This is called a bronchoprovocation (brong-KO-prav-eh-KA-shun) test. Using spirometry, this test repeatedly measures your lung function

during physical activity or after you receive increasing doses of cold air or a special chemical to breathe in.

- A test to show whether you have another condition with the same symptoms as asthma, such as reflux disease, vocal cord dysfunction, or sleep apnea.
- A <u>chest x ray</u> or an <u>EKG</u> (electrocardiogram). These tests will help find out whether a foreign object or other disease may be causing your symptoms.

Diagnosing Asthma in Young Children

Most children who have asthma develop their first symptoms before 5 years of age. However, asthma in young children (aged 0 to 5 years) can be hard to diagnose.

Sometimes it's hard to tell whether a child has asthma or another childhood condition. This is because the symptoms of asthma also occur with other conditions.

Also, many young children who wheeze when they get colds or respiratory infections don't go on to have asthma after they're 6 years old.

A child may wheeze because he or she has small airways that become even narrower during colds or respiratory infections. The airways grow as the child grows older, so wheezing no longer occurs when the child gets colds.

A young child who has frequent wheezing with colds or respiratory infections is more likely to have asthma if:

- One or both parents have asthma
- The child has signs of allergies, including the allergic skin condition eczema
- The child has allergic reactions to pollens or other airborne allergens
- The child wheezes even when he or she doesn't have a cold or other infection

The most certain way to diagnose asthma is with a lung function test, a medical history, and a physical exam. However, it's hard to do lung function tests in children younger than 5 years. Thus, doctors must rely on children's medical histories, signs and symptoms, and physical exams to make a diagnosis.

Doctors also may use a 4–6 week trial of asthma medicines to see how well a child responds.

How Is Asthma Treated and Controlled?

Asthma is a long-term disease that has no cure. The goal of asthma treatment is to control the disease. Good asthma control will:

- Prevent chronic and troublesome symptoms, such as <u>coughing</u> and shortness of breath
- Reduce your need for quick-relief medicines (see below)
- Help you maintain good lung function
- Let you maintain your normal activity level and sleep through the night
- Prevent asthma attacks that could result in an emergency room visit or hospital stay

To control asthma, partner with your doctor to manage your asthma or your child's asthma. Children aged 10 or older—and younger children who are able—should take an active role in their asthma care.

Taking an active role to control your asthma involves:

- Working with your doctor to treat other conditions that can interfere with asthma management.
- Avoiding things that worsen your asthma (asthma triggers). However, one trigger you should not avoid is physical activity. Physical activity is an important part of a healthy lifestyle. Talk with your doctor about medicines that can help you stay active.

- Working with your doctor and other health care providers to create and follow an asthma action plan.

An asthma action plan gives guidance on taking your medicines properly, avoiding asthma triggers (except physical activity), tracking your level of asthma control, responding to worsening symptoms, and seeking emergency care when needed.

Asthma is treated with two types of medicines: long-term control and quick-relief medicines. Long-term control medicines help reduce airway inflammation and prevent asthma symptoms. Quick-relief, or "rescue," medicines relieve asthma symptoms that may flare up.

Your initial treatment will depend on the severity of your asthma. Followup asthma treatment will depend on how well your asthma action plan is controlling your symptoms and preventing asthma attacks.

Your level of asthma control can vary over time and with changes in your home, school, or work environments. These changes can alter how often you're exposed to the factors that can worsen your asthma.

Your doctor may need to increase your medicine if your asthma doesn't stay under control. On the other hand, if your asthma is well controlled for several months, your doctor may decrease your medicine. These adjustments to your medicine will help you maintain the best control possible with the least amount of medicine necessary.

Asthma treatment for certain groups of people—such as children, pregnant women, or those for whom exercise brings on asthma symptoms—will be adjusted to meet their special needs.

Follow an Asthma Action Plan

You can work with your doctor to create a personal asthma action plan. The plan will describe your daily treatments, such as which medicines to take and when to take them. The plan also will explain when to call your doctor or go to the emergency room.

If your child has asthma, all of the people who care for him or her should know about the child's asthma action plan. This includes babysitters and workers at daycare centers, schools, and camps. These caretakers can help your child follow his or her action plan.

Avoid Things That Can Worsen Your Asthma

Many common things (called asthma triggers) can set off or worsen your asthma symptoms. Once you know what these things are, you can take steps to control many of them.

For example, exposure to pollens or air pollution might make your asthma worse. If so, try to limit time outdoors when the levels of these substances in the outdoor air are high. If animal fur triggers your asthma symptoms, keep pets with fur out of your home or bedroom.

One possible asthma trigger you shouldn't avoid is physical activity. Physical activity is an important part of a healthy lifestyle. Talk with your doctor about medicines that can help you stay active.

If your asthma symptoms are clearly related to allergens, and you can't avoid exposure to those allergens, your doctor may advise you to get allergy shots.

You may need to see a specialist if you're thinking about getting allergy shots. These shots can lessen or prevent your asthma symptoms, but they can't cure your asthma.

Several health conditions can make asthma harder to manage. These conditions include runny nose, sinus infections, reflux disease, psychological stress, and <u>sleep apnea</u>. Your doctor will treat these conditions as well.

Medicines

Your doctor will consider many things when deciding which asthma medicines are best for you. He or she will check to see how well a medicine works for you. Then, he or she will adjust the dose or medicine as needed.

Asthma medicines can be taken in pill form, but most are taken using a device called an inhaler. An inhaler allows the medicine to go directly to your lungs.

Not all inhalers are used the same way. Ask your doctor or another health care provider to show you the right way to use your inhaler. Review the way you use your inhaler at every medical visit.

Long-Term Control Medicines

Most people who have asthma need to take long-term control medicines daily to help prevent symptoms. The most effective long-term medicines reduce airway inflammation, which helps prevent symptoms from starting. These medicines don't give you quick relief from symptoms.

Inhaled corticosteroids. Inhaled corticosteroids are the preferred medicine for long-term control of asthma. They're the most effective option for long-term relief of the inflammation and swelling that makes your airways sensitive to certain inhaled substances.

Reducing inflammation helps prevent the chain reaction that causes asthma symptoms. Most people who take these medicines daily find they greatly reduce the severity of symptoms and how often they occur.

Inhaled corticosteroids generally are safe when taken as prescribed. These medicines are different from the illegal anabolic steroids taken by some athletes. Inhaled corticosteroids aren't habit-forming, even if you take them every day for many years.

Like many other medicines, though, inhaled corticosteroids can have side effects. Most doctors agree that the benefits of taking inhaled corticosteroids and preventing asthma attacks far outweigh the risk of side effects.

One common side effect from inhaled corticosteroids is a mouth infection called thrush. You might be able to use a spacer or holding chamber on your inhaler to avoid thrush. These devices attach to your inhaler. They help prevent the medicine from landing in your mouth or on the back of your throat.

Check with your doctor to see whether a spacer or holding chamber should be used with the inhaler you have. Also, work with your health care team if you have any questions about how to use a spacer or holding chamber. Rinsing your mouth out with water after taking inhaled corticosteroids also can lower your risk for thrush.

If you have severe asthma, you may have to take corticosteroid pills or liquid for short periods to get your asthma under control.

If taken for long periods, these medicines raise your risk for cataracts and osteoporosis (OS-te-o-po-RO-sis). A cataract is the clouding of the lens in your eye. Osteoporosis is a disorder that makes your bones weak and more likely to break.

Your doctor may have you add another long-term asthma control medicine so he or she can lower your dose of corticosteroids. Or, your doctor may suggest you take calcium and vitamin D pills to protect your bones.

Other long-term control medicines. Other long-term control medicines include:

- <u>Cromolyn</u>. This medicine is taken using a device called a nebulizer. As you breathe in, the nebulizer sends a fine mist of medicine to your lungs. Cromolyn helps prevent airway inflammation.
- <u>Omalizumab</u> (anti-IgE). This medicine is given as a shot (injection) one or two times a month. It helps prevent your body from reacting to asthma triggers, such as pollen and dust mites. Anti-IgE might be used if other asthma medicines have not worked well.

A rare, but possibly life-threatening allergic reaction called anaphylaxis might occur when the Omalizumab injection is given. If you take this medication, work with your doctor to make sure you understand the signs and symptoms of anaphylaxis and what actions you should take.

- <u>Inhaled long-acting beta2-agonists</u>. These medicines open the airways. They might be added to inhaled corticosteroids to improve asthma control. Inhaled long-acting beta2-agonists should never be used on their own for long-term asthma control. They must used with inhaled corticosteroids.
- <u>Leukotriene modifiers</u>. These medicines are taken by mouth. They help block the chain reaction that increases inflammation in your airways.

- <u>Theophylline</u>. This medicine is taken by mouth. Theophylline helps open the airways.

If your doctor prescribes a long-term control medicine, take it every day to control your asthma. Your asthma symptoms will likely return or get worse if you stop taking your medicine.

Long-term control medicines can have side effects. Talk with your doctor about these side effects and ways to reduce or avoid them.

With some medicines, like theophylline, your doctor will check the level of medicine in your blood. This helps ensure that you're getting enough medicine to relieve your asthma symptoms, but not so much that it causes dangerous side effects.

Quick-Relief Medicines

All people who have asthma need quick-relief medicines to help relieve asthma symptoms that may flare up. <u>Inhaled short-acting beta2-agonists</u> are the first choice for quick relief.

These medicines act quickly to relax tight muscles around your airways when you're having a flareup. This allows the airways to open up so air can flow through them.

You should take your quick-relief medicine when you first notice asthma symptoms. If you use this medicine more than 2 days a week, talk with your doctor about your asthma control. You may need to make changes to your asthma action plan.

Carry your quick-relief inhaler with you at all times in case you need it. If your child has asthma, make sure that anyone caring for him or her has the child's quick-relief medicines, including staff at the child's school. They should understand when and how to use these medicines and when to seek medical care for your child.

You shouldn't use quick-relief medicines in place of prescribed long-term control medicines. Quick-relief medicines don't reduce inflammation.

Track Your Asthma

To track your asthma, keep records of your symptoms, check your peak flow number using a peak flow meter, and get regular asthma checkups.

Record Your Symptoms

You can record your asthma symptoms in a diary to see how well your treatments are controlling your asthma.

Asthma is well controlled if:

- You have symptoms no more than 2 days a week, and these symptoms don't wake you from sleep more than 1 or 2 nights a month.
- You can do all your normal activities.
- You take quick-relief medicines no more than 2 days a week.
- You have no more than one asthma attack a year that requires you to take corticosteroids by mouth.
- Your peak flow doesn't drop below 80 percent of your personal best number.

If your asthma isn't well controlled, contact your doctor. He or she may need to change your asthma action plan.

Use a Peak Flow Meter

This small, hand-held device shows how well air moves out of your lungs. You blow into the device and it gives you a score, or peak flow number. Your score shows how well your lungs are working at the time of the test.

Your doctor will tell you how and when to use your peak flow meter. He or she also will teach you how to take your medicines based on your score.

Your doctor and other health care providers may ask you to use your peak flow meter each morning and keep a record of your results. You may find it very useful to record peak flow scores for a couple of weeks before each medical visit and take the results with you.

When you're first diagnosed with asthma, it's important to find your "personal best" peak flow number. To do this, you record your score each day for a 2- to 3-week period when your asthma is well-controlled. The highest number you get during that time is your personal best. You can compare this number to future numbers to make sure your asthma is controlled.

Your peak flow meter can help warn you of an asthma attack, even before you notice symptoms. If your score shows that your breathing is getting worse, you should take your quick-relief medicines the way your asthma action plan directs. Then you can use the peak flow meter to check how well the medicine worked.

Get Asthma Checkups

When you first begin treatment, you'll see your doctor about every 2 to 6 weeks. Once your asthma is controlled, your doctor may want to see you from once a month to twice a year.

During these checkups, your doctor may ask whether you've had an asthma attack since the last visit or any changes in symptoms or peak flow measurements. He or she also may ask about your daily activities. This information will help your doctor assess your level of asthma control.

Your doctor also may ask whether you have any problems or concerns with taking your medicines or following your asthma action plan. Based on your answers to these questions, your doctor may change the dose of your medicine or give you a new medicine.

If your control is very good, you might be able to take less medicine. The goal is to use the least amount of medicine needed to control your asthma.

Emergency Care

Most people who have asthma, including many children, can safely manage their symptoms by following their asthma action plans. However, you might need medical attention at times.

Call your doctor for advice if:

- Your medicines don't relieve an asthma attack.
- Your peak flow is less than half of your personal best peak flow number.

Call 9–1–1 for emergency care if:

- You have trouble walking and talking because you're out of breath.
- You have blue lips or fingernails.

At the hospital, you'll be closely watched and given <u>oxygen</u> and more medicines, as well as medicines at higher doses than you take at home. Such treatment can save your life.

Asthma Treatment for Special Groups

The treatments described above generally apply to all people who have asthma. However, some aspects of treatment differ for people in certain age groups and those who have special needs.

Children

It's hard to diagnose asthma in children younger than 5 years. Thus, it's hard to know whether young children who wheeze or have other asthma symptoms will benefit from long-term control medicines. (Quick-relief medicines tend to relieve wheezing in young children whether they have asthma or not.)

Doctors will treat infants and young children who have asthma symptoms with long-term control medicines if, after assessing a child, they feel that the symptoms are persistent and likely to continue after 6 years of age.

Inhaled corticosteroids are the preferred treatment for young children. Montelukast and cromolyn are other options. Treatment might be given for a trial period of 1 month to 6 weeks. Treatment usually is stopped if benefits aren't seen during that time and the doctor and parents are confident the medicine was used properly.

Inhaled corticosteroids can possibly slow the growth of children of all ages. Slowed growth usually is apparent in the first several months of treatment, is generally small, and doesn't get worse over time. Poorly controlled asthma also may reduce a child's growth rate.

Many experts think the benefits of inhaled corticosteroids for children who need them to control their asthma far outweigh the risk of slowed growth.

Older Adults

Doctors may need to adjust asthma treatment for older adults who take certain other medicines, such as beta blockers, aspirin and other pain relievers, and anti-inflammatory medicines. These medicines can prevent asthma medicines from working well and may worsen asthma symptoms.

Be sure to tell your doctor about all of the medicines you take, including over-the-counter medicines.

Older adults may develop weak bones from using inhaled corticosteroids, especially at high doses. Talk with your doctor about taking calcium and vitamin D pills, as well as other ways to help keep your bones strong.

Pregnant Women

Pregnant women who have asthma need to control the disease to ensure a good supply of oxygen to their babies. Poor asthma control increases the risk of preeclampsia, a condition in which a pregnant woman develops high blood pressure and protein in the urine. Poor asthma control also increases the risk that a baby will be born early and have a low birth weight.

Studies show that it's safer to take asthma medicines while pregnant than to risk having an asthma attack.

Talk with your doctor if you have asthma and are pregnant or planning a pregnancy. Your level of asthma control may get better or it may get worse while you're pregnant. Your health care team will check your asthma control often and adjust your treatment as needed.

People Whose Asthma Symptoms Occur With Physical Activity

Physical activity is an important part of a healthy lifestyle. Adults need physical activity to maintain good health. Children need it for growth and development.

In some people, however, physical activity can trigger asthma symptoms. If this happens to you or your child, talk with your doctor about the best ways to control asthma so you can stay active.

The following medicines may help prevent asthma symptoms caused by physical activity:

- Short-acting beta2-agonists (quick-relief medicine) taken shortly before physical activity can last 2 to 3 hours and prevent exercise-related symptoms in most people who take them.
- Long-acting beta2-agonists can be protective for up to 12 hours. However, with daily use, they'll no longer give up to 12 hours of protection. Also, frequent use of these medicines for physical activity might be a sign that asthma is poorly controlled.

- Leukotriene modifiers. These pills are taken several hours before physical activity. They can help relieve asthma symptoms brought on by physical activity.
- Long-term control medicines. Frequent or severe symptoms due to physical activity may suggest poorly controlled asthma and the need to either start or increase long-term control medicines that reduce inflammation. This will help prevent exercise-related symptoms.

Easing into physical activity with a warmup period may be helpful. You also may want to wear a mask or scarf over your mouth when exercising in cold weather.

If you use your asthma medicines as your doctor directs, you should be able to take part in any physical activity or sport you choose.

People Having Surgery

Asthma may add to the risk of having problems during and after surgery. For instance, having a tube put into your throat may cause an asthma attack.

Tell your surgeon about your asthma when you first talk with him or her. The surgeon can take steps to lower your risk, such as giving you asthma medicines before or during surgery.

How Can Asthma Be Prevented?

You can't prevent asthma. However, you can take steps to control the disease and prevent its symptoms. For example:

- Learn about your asthma and ways to control it.
- Follow your written asthma action plan.
- Use medicines as your doctor prescribes.
- Identify and try to avoid things that make your asthma worse (asthma triggers). However, one trigger you should not avoid is physical activity. Physical activity is an important part of a healthy lifestyle. Talk with your doctor about medicines that can help you stay active.
- Keep track of your asthma symptoms and level of control.
- Get regular checkups for your asthma.

Living With Asthma

If you have asthma, you'll need long-term care. Successful asthma treatment requires that you take an active role in your care and follow your asthma action plan.

Learn How To Manage Your Asthma

Partner with your doctor to develop an asthma action plan. This plan will help you know when and how to take your medicines. The plan also will help you identify your asthma triggers and manage your disease if asthma symptoms worsen.

Children aged 10 or older—and younger children who can handle it—should be involved in creating and following their asthma action plans.

Most people who have asthma can successfully manage their symptoms by following their asthma action plans and having regular checkups. However, knowing when to seek emergency medical care is important.

Learn how to use your medicines correctly. If you take inhaled medicines, you should practice using your inhaler at your doctor's office. If you take long-term control medicines, take them daily as your doctor prescribes.

Record your asthma symptoms as a way to track how well your asthma is controlled. Also, your doctor may advise you to use a peak flow meter to measure and record how well your lungs are working.

Your doctor may ask you to keep records of your symptoms or peak flow results daily for a couple of weeks before an office visit. You'll bring these records with you to the visit.

These steps will help you keep track of how well you're controlling your asthma over time. This will help you spot problems early and prevent or relieve asthma attacks. Recording your symptoms and peak flow results to share with your doctor also will help him or her decide whether to adjust your treatment.

Ongoing Care

Have regular asthma checkups with your doctor so he or she can assess your level of asthma control and adjust your treatment as needed. Remember, the main goal of asthma treatment is to achieve the best control of your asthma using the least amount of medicine. This may require frequent adjustments to your treatments.

If you find it hard to follow your asthma action plan or the plan isn't working well, let your health care team know right away. They will work with you to adjust your plan to better suit your needs.

Get treatment for any other conditions that can interfere with your asthma management.

Watch for Signs That Your Asthma Is Getting Worse

Your asthma might be getting worse if:

- Your symptoms start to occur more often, are more severe, or bother you at night and cause you to lose sleep.
- You're limiting your normal activities and missing school or work because of your asthma.
- Your peak flow number is low compared to your personal best or varies a lot from day to day.
- Your asthma medicines don't seem to work well anymore.
- You have to use your quick-relief inhaler more often. If you're using quick-relief medicine more than 2 days a week, your asthma isn't well controlled.
- You have to go to the emergency room or doctor because of an asthma attack.

If you have any of these signs, see your doctor. He or she might need to change your medicines or take other steps to control your asthma.

Partner with your health care team and take an active role in your care. This can help you better control your asthma so it doesn't interfere with your activities and disrupt your life.

2. 314 Great Tips For Getting Quick Relief From Asthma

Asthma is a serious problem that millions of people suffer around the world. If your asthma medication isn't working, or isn't as effective as you'd like it to be, then follow these simple tips in this book to help relieve and lessen the symptoms and help you lead a healthy, enjoyable life.

1. Buy a dehumidifier if you suffer from seasonal allergies. Dry environments are much better for asthmatics than high humidity areas. The use of a dehumidifier will create the best home for your asthma issues. Doing so will help out the entire family as well since the house will be more pleasant to live in.

2. If you enjoy using a vaporizer or a humidifier, you have to make sure it is clean before each use. These types of machines can build up a lot of dust and calcium, that you do not want getting into the air you breath. You need to be breathing the cleanest air possible, at all times.

3. There is help for when you feel an asthma attack coming on and your inhaler is not with you. Caffeinated drinks can help you as they open your airways. Drink a couple of cups of coffee, tea, or hot chocolate before the full onset of your attack to minimize its negative effects.

4. Keep your stress level as low as humanly possible. As anxiety levels increase due to everyday problems, so do asthma symptoms. If you experience wheezing and coughing several times a day, consider stress relief techniques such as regular exercises and stretching and breathing exercises. Also, be sure you get enough sleep to deal with the stresses of everyday life.

5. Try to reduce the amount of environmental allergens and pollutants, such as dust, pollens, pet hair, molds and fungi, and food particles. Keeping your house clean can make a huge difference for your asthma symptoms. Buying an air filter or purifier, or even cleaning out the filters in your AC system can also help.

6. To cut the risk of an asthma attack, keep your house as clean as you can, particularly the bedroom of the person with asthma. Food should be eaten only in the kitchen or dining room, and cigarettes are best relegated to

outdoor smoking areas. After cleaning around the house, open windows and allow fresh air into the house. This can reduce the smell and pervasiveness of household cleaners like bleach.

7. Pay attention to your attack triggers. If you know what is likely to trigger your attacks, such as smoke, animals, or pollen, then you can make a better effort to avoid them. Asthma triggers are different for everyone. Unfortunately, the only real way to know what will trigger an attack is to have one, and then remember what happened.

8. Household plants and flowers can act as an asthma attack trigger. The reason for this is that many of them carry pollen and other particles that can get into the air. They can cause problems even if the air is well circulated in the home. To be completely safe, don't bring plants and flowers into the home, and if someone has them delivered to your home, throw them out immediately.

9. Smoke is one of the worst asthma aggravators. It goes without saying that asthma sufferers should not smoke, but some consideration on the part of those they live with is called for, too. A household that includes an asthma sufferer must be a smoke-free one. Smokers in the household

must be willing to keep the indoor air clean out of medical necessity.

10. When you are near or at a gas station make sure that your windows are always rolled up. Gasoline gives off very strong fumes which can impact the quality of the air around you and worsen your asthma. Reduce your interaction with gas stations to allow for quality air intake.

11. It is important to remain positive and optimistic as much as possible. Stress and worry can cause asthma symptoms to flare up, Make sure you try to keep your daily life balanced and stress free as much as possible. There will always be things that cause stress, but it is just important to do what you can to minimize stress and worry.

12. If you have a child who suffers from asthma, make sure that you educate him about asthma and why following his treatment plans are so important. You should not only discuss what to do when he suffers an attack, you should also act out the steps. This will help your child to stay calm during an attack. Make sure that you also educate caregivers and siblings.

13. Be prepared in case of an asthma emergency. Locate the nearest emergency room to your

home and have your asthma action plan and the medications you are taking written down to take with you. Be sure to note the dosages and purposes of each. Have an emergency contact on hand who can take care of watching your children or other necessities if you should have to go to the ER.

14. By using a peak flow meter to measure the strength of your breaths, you can sometimes recognize an asthma attack coming on long before you actually feel the symptoms. That's why it's good to have a peak flow meter and use it frequently throughout the day. Be sure to establish your normal reading at an optimum time so you will have a point of comparison.

15. You can recognize asthma by its symptoms, such as wheezing, shallow breathing, tightness in the chest and coughing. An asthma attack may be triggered by a wide variety of things. Among them are anxiety, acid reflux, some kinds of food and/or medicines, heavy exercise, contact with irritants and allergens, the common cold, or a sinus infection.

16. A great tip that can help you get a grip on your asthma is to bring your own pillow when you travel anywhere. You never know how much

dust there's going to be when you're staying at different places. Bringing your own clean pillow will reduce the risk of breathing in dust.

17. When it is humid outside, it is best for asthma sufferers to remain indoors. The pollen count is high during high humidity, and that can cause an asthma flare up. It is also a good idea to stay inside when the seasons are changing for the same reasons as the humidity.

18. If you have asthma, know your triggers. What is it that causes an asthma attack to come on? Many common triggers are allergies and irritants. For some, it is exercise or extreme temperatures. Emotional or anxiety issues can also cause asthma type attacks. Knowing what causes your attack can also be what will help you find a proper treatment.

19. Keeping yourself healthy can be a way to control your asthma better. The common cold, as well as viruses and bacterial infections can cause a flare up or attack of your asthma. Especially colds which produce mucus or a nasal drip that can end up in your lungs.

20. Be sure you understand how to use the medication you're given for asthma properly,

especially your rescue medication. Asthma is a condition traditionally treated with a combination of a regular medicine and an emergency medicinal inhaler. Asthma is an illness that is chronic in nature, so it is imperative to take the management medicine as directed and only using the rescue inhaler when necessary.

21. Know what triggers your asthma and how to avoid them. Triggers are different for each person, so it may take some time to figure out what yours are. Keep a diary of them. Once you find out what your triggers are, try to avoid or limit your contact with them.

22. Be your child's asthma advocate, especially at school. Many schools have policies in place that prohibit children from carrying medications on them. This is not acceptable when it comes to an emergency rescue inhaler. Find out what steps you need to take to make sure that your child has access to their medication as needed.

23. Find some relaxation techniques that work for you to help you when you notice an oncoming asthma attack. Options such as deep breathing, imagery, muscle relaxation and meditation can help you calm your breathing and reduce stress levels, helping you get control of worsening

symptoms, especially those caused by stress or anxiety.

24. Take note of how often, from a weekly standpoint, you use the rescue inhaler. If the inhaler is used more than twice, the asthma problems you are suffering from may not be well-managed or something else might be causing additional attacks to come on. You can use your frequency of inhaler use to gauge the effectiveness of your asthma treatment plan and make modifications when necessary.

25. If you are struggling with asthma, you should cover your mattresses and pillows with plastic covers. Mattresses and pillows can trap in many triggers for asthma attacks, such as dust and dirt. You should try to wash your bedding once a week in hot water to remove the build up on asthma triggers.

26. To decrease your asthma symptoms, you should try to avoid going outside during humid seasons. You should also try to stay inside when the seasons are changing. The amount of pollen in the air increases with a season change. Pollen is one of the main triggers for asthma attacks and other asthma symptoms.

27. If you are prone to attacks during allergy season, make use of over the counter allergy medications. While allergies and asthma are not the same, they do have many of the same mechanisms, and many people have both seasonal allergies and asthma. A seasonal allergy attack can compound the effects of asthma.

28. Wash your bedding, including your pillowcases, at least weekly, using hot water and chlorinated bleach. This will be more effective at killing dust mites than the use of liquid washing detergent alone. You have to wash bedding regularly to prevent the ones that do survive from continuing to multiply and causing problems.

29. When it comes to asthma, many people have been known to abuse their inhalers without even realizing it. It is not a breath freshener, it is only to be used when you have a serious attack. Sometimes just simple calming breathing techniques or stopping moving are all you need to stop an attack. Don't always resort to your inhaler as this can make your body stop reacting to it and make it useless.

30. If asthma is really severely impacting your life consider joining a support group for asthma sufferers. This will help you know that you are

not alone. Often times feeling alone you may become depressed in unable to follow doctors instructions, and, or, keep doctors appointments. As such the quality of your care will go down. A support group will help prevent this.

31. The first thing to do when you find out you have asthma is to find out if you also have allergies. Have your doctor perform a skin test to see if you are allergic to some of the common allergens such as dust, dander, pollen, and so on that can aggravate your asthma.

32. You might think that using a fan will help you breathe better. If you do not dust your house properly, using a fan will cause the air to carry dust particles. This may cause you to experience difficulties breathing. You should always dust your house before you use a fan.

33. If you're caught without your inhaler when you have an attack, grab a cup of coffee. The caffeine in the beverage will open up your airways and allow you to breathe a little easier. If you don't have a caffeinated beverage on hand, the small amounts of caffeine in a chocolate bar can also help.

34. Learn how to recognize asthma so you can treat it. When you get asthma, you usually have difficulties breathing and feel as if your chest were getting tighter. Asthma is often accompanied by coughing and wheezing. If you experience different symptoms, you might have another illness that requires more medical attention.

35. If you suffer from asthma, it is crucial that you are using your inhaler properly. Make sure that you take a deep breath before taking your asthma pump. By not using your asthma inhaler properly, you may not be getting the proper treatment in order to control your asthma symptoms.

36. Get a bronchodilator or an inhaler. These products usually allow you to breathe better a few seconds after you use them. There are risks inherent to using these products, but if you use them as prescribed they should make your life easier. Ask your doctor about what kind of inhaler you should use.

37. Keep your bed linens washed on at least a weekly basis. Make sure to always wash them in hot water. This will keep your bed from harboring dust mites and other allergens that can

trigger an attack. Having as clean a home as possible is one of the best defenses against asthma.

38. You may want to get into a support group if you have asthma. The people in the group are in the same situation as you so they know what you have to go through everyday. Also, they may have personal tips of what you can do to control your asthma symptoms.

39. Make sure you know your breathing. Observe the way you breathe when you are calm and symptom free. When you realize that your breathing has changed you can consider relaxation and breathing techniques to calm you down to avoid severe asthma attacks. During an attack, try to return your breathing to its normal depth and rate.

40. If you have asthma and you are going to be traveling by air, be sure to get a note from your doctor stating your condition and what medications you take. Airports are picky on what can be brought on board, but asthma patients are always permitted to bring medications and inhalers on board, as long as they have a doctor's note.

41. Be sure to take plenty of Vitamins C and E if you have asthma. These particular vitamins are believed to better your lung function and help manage your symptoms of asthma. You are able to get these vitamins either from food or a supplement. The vitamins can help to boost the immune system, which will help you to stay healthy and less ill, which means you will have less asthma attacks.

42. IF you have asthma, you should consider buying a dehumidifier. Dust mites are a major source of asthma attacks, and dehumidifiers are great at getting rid of the little buggers. Try running a dehumidifier to dry up the air in your home.

43. Stay indoors when grass is being mown or clipped if grass pollen is one of your asthma triggers. Because lawn care stirs up the pollen, being in the vicinity when the grass is being cut can cause an asthma attack. Instead, remain indoors with the windows and doors closed to lessen your exposure to the pollen.

44. Keep track of upcoming weather conditions that may affect your asthma. Some sufferers are affected more strongly than others by changes in barometric pressure or humidity. If you are one of these, being aware of upcoming storms or

changes in weather to help you find ways to manage the changes in weather to limit the impact on your asthma symptoms.

45. You may want to consider having numerous doctors treat your asthma. Your usual doctor will be able to help you, but you should also consider seeing a specialist. Asthma doctors, allergists, and pulmiologists are the people who you want to consult with to help with asthma.

46. Those with asthma should remain inside as much as they can when the pollen count rises. The same pollens and other irritants that cause trouble for allergy sufferers are also concerns for asthma sufferers, even though the two are quite distinct conditions. Information about local air quality is available in many areas so that those with asthma can reduce their outdoor exposure if irritants are within the air.

47. It is important to stay indoors during certain seasons when you have asthma. Some times of the year when the air is especially humid, spending too much time outdoors can make it difficult for you to breathe. Other times, the pollen count gets very high and can trigger an asthma attack.

48. If inhaler use happens more than two times in each of your weeks, you must schedule an appointment with your doctor about this and possibly adjust your medication. This might mean that your inhaler isn't working enough for you. This also applies to anyone who needs to refill their inhaler more than two times in a single year.

49. If you suffer from asthma, it is crucial that you are using your inhaler properly. Make sure that you take a deep breath before taking your asthma pump. By not using your asthma inhaler properly, you may not be getting the proper treatment in order to control your asthma symptoms.

50. Keep your bed linens washed on at least a weekly basis. Make sure to always wash them in hot water. This will keep your bed from harboring dust mites and other allergens that can trigger an attack. Having as clean a home as possible is one of the best defenses against asthma.

51. Let your friends know that they should not give you gifts of household plants. Plants can be a severe trigger for certain asthmatics. Having them constantly in your home would be like

fighting a war with your environment every day. If someone does give you a plant, see if it can be planted outside. If it can't be moved outdoors, thank them nicely for the gift and then give it away later.

52. Medications that will help you control symptoms when you have an attack are oral corticosteroids and bronchodilators. Bronchodilators, usually referred to as "rescue medications", are usually inhaled but also come in liquid, tablet, or they are injectable. These are the most popular forms of 'rescue medications' that you can get.

53. Leukotriene inhibitors are a very popular treatment for people that have asthma. This type of medication will work to stop chemical substances that can cause an asthma attack. It is very important that if you are prescribed these, you make sure to take it exactly how your doctor tells you to.

54. An annual flu vaccination is highly recommended for yourself and your family. If you have asthma, you can protect your health by taking all steps possible to avoid any type of cold, flu or other upper respiratory infection. The easiest way to start is by performing routine

hand-washing, limiting your touching of surfaces while in public places, and getting vaccinations recommended by your doctor.

55. Be careful when starting an exercise program, and always ease into strenuous activities. Physical exertion isn't an asthma trigger for everyone, but all asthmatics suffer from some degree of airway constriction all the time, by definition, which makes it harder on your system when you work out. For those whose asthma is triggered by exercise, easing in can make it possible to exercise without suffering an attack.

56. If tobacco smoke is a trigger for your asthma symptoms, not only should you not smoke, but you should also avoid places where people smoke. Tobacco smoke leaves a film behind, so even if there is no fresh smoke in the air, the chemicals left behind may still trigger an asthma attack.

57. Make sure you use your preventative inhaler that is prescribed by your doctor. Note that a preventative inhaler is different than a rescue inhaler, which is used during an acute attack. A preventative inhaler, on the other hand, dispenses medicine designed to keep the air flowing, which reduces acute attacks.

58. If you have asthma, you should avoid places that have high levels of dust. Dust can cause an asthma attack very easily. Some places that have high dust levels are attics, basements, and unoccupied homes that have been unoccupied for a period of time. If you must go into a dusty area, do not use any fans. The fans will spread the dust around you.

59. The homes of asthma sufferers should be inspected thoroughly and regularly for mold, dust and spores. People who suffer from asthma are particularly susceptible to the kinds of allergens and airborne particulates that can cause respiratory trouble. A professional inspection can identify these asthma aggravators and pinpoint their sources for removal.

60. Any allergy can have a deleterious synergy with an asthma condition, and food allergies are no different. If you have asthma problems, a clinical food allergy test can help you pinpoint problem foods. A mild food allergy could exacerbate your asthma without your noticing. A full medical test can help you identify foods you need to avoid to keep your asthma in check.

61. You may think using fans indoors would be a good thing to help reduce your asthma symptoms. However, if there is any amount of dust in the area and the space is closed up, using a fan is only going to kick that dust up into the air that your breathe. This could trigger an asthma attack, so avoid using fans in closed up, dusty places.

62. Find out as much as possible about your condition. The more educated you are about your asthma, the more proactive you can be about your treatment. Keep up with trends and new treatment methods, and ensure that the medical professionals on your team are working hard to help you. The best thing to do is learn and research as much as you can about this condition and the treatment options that would be best for you.

63. If you are affected with asthma, stay away from men or women who wear very strong colognes or perfumes. These scents can tarnish the quality of the air you're breathing, and can lead to shortness of breath. Additionally, you should try to limit the amount of body sprays that you put on your skin in the morning and evening.

64. Take care of your body from the inside out to avoid getting sick. When you get sick, you will have a lot of trouble breathing, which can exacerbate your asthma symptoms. In the morning, consume various fruits that contain a high dose of vitamin C to prevent from getting colds.

65. If you're caught without your inhaler when you have an attack, grab a cup of coffee. The caffeine in the beverage will open up your airways and allow you to breathe a little easier. If you don't have a caffeinated beverage on hand, the small amounts of caffeine in a chocolate bar can also help.

66. A great tip that can help you alleviate your asthma is to make sure you're properly using your inhaler. A lot of people don't use their inhaler correctly because they take shallow breaths. In order for the medicine to work, you need to inhale deeply when using your inhaler.

67. Avoid anything that could trigger your asthma. This could be something you're allergic to like pollen or dust. Others may need to avoid certain physical activities to keep from suffering an attack. Keep a journal of your attacks so that you

can start to learn what your triggers are so that you can prevent flareups before they begin.

68. Beta 2 antagonists that can be inhaled are long term asthma control medicines that can be taken every day. They may also have risks for certain people as well. When you are taking these medications it is now recommended they be used along with corticosteroids that can be inhaled.

69. Use natural remedies for your asthma. While doctor-prescribed medication might be necessary to prevent deadly attacks, a healthy diet will help to improve everyday life. Beta carotene's promote healthy mucus membranes in your mouth and nose which help to reduce the chances of serious asthma attacks.

70. To alleviate or prevent asthma attacks, minimize how often and much you come into contact with animals. Even if you are not allergic to pet hair or dander, a common occurrence with asthma, you can have an attack triggered by the dirt or pet dander simply being in the air. If you have pets in the home, vacuum often to limit pet-triggered air pollutants.

71. You will need to keep your residence really clean, especially the bedroom where the asthma

sufferer sleeps in order to help lessen the chances of an attack. Food should be restricted to the kitchen, and smoking inside the home should never be permitted. Bypass chemicals when cleaning your home if at all possible, and be sure to open doors and windows afterwards.

72. A yearly home inspection by a qualified professional for common asthma triggers, such as mold spores and dust, is a must for asthma sufferers. Removing any of these substance's if they are present in your home can reduce the number of asthma attacks suffered and make life more comfortable for the entire family.

73. Invest in a dehumidifier if you have an asthma sufferer in your home. A dry environment is the most comfortable for those with asthma and lessens the likelihood of an attack. A dry environment also discourages the growth of mold and spores, which are common asthma triggers for many individuals.

74. For temporary relief of asthma symptoms there are quick-relief medications. They are oral corticosteroids and bronchodilators. Bronchodilators are often called rescue medication and open up airways and allow more air to flow through. Corticosteroids are designed

for short-term use and are either swallowed or given by injection. They work by treating inflammation in airways.

75. When traveling by air, keep all of your asthma medications in your carry-on, and put this bag under the seat in front of you. This ensures that the staff will be unable to lose your medications. It also gives you access to your meds during times when you can't get into the overhead bins, such as during take-off and landing.

76. Find some relaxation techniques that work for you to help you when you notice an oncoming asthma attack. Options such as deep breathing, imagery, muscle relaxation and meditation can help you calm your breathing and reduce stress levels, helping you get control of worsening symptoms, especially those caused by stress or anxiety.

77. To decrease your asthma symptoms, you should try to avoid going outside during humid seasons. You should also try to stay inside when the seasons are changing. The amount of pollen in the air increases with a season change. Pollen is one of the main triggers for asthma attacks and other asthma symptoms.

78. A dehumidifier can help ease your asthma symptoms. The wettest season is typically the season when you experience the worst asthma aggravation. A dehumidifier can make your home a pleasant refuge from seasonal asthma triggers. Dry air is easier for the asthma sufferer to breathe. You should always ensure that the dehumidifier you use - like all air-treatment devices - is clean before using it.

79. If you have asthma, it is important to avoid allergens. These irritants can trigger an attack and cause coughing, wheezing and shortness of breath. Things you should stay away from are tobacco smoke, pollen, dust, mold and pet dander. Some people are also sensitive to cold air or overexerting themselves.

80. Learn all that you can learn about the condition you have. Having the right information can enable you to choose the treatments that are right for you, and help reduce symptoms. Do your research, and keep current on available treatment information so you can be sure you're doing all you can to feel well. You need to learn about asthma and the treatment options available.

81. Controlling your asthma is sometimes a hard thing to do. If you are finding yourself using your quick relief inhaler more than twice a week than something needs to be done. You may want to consider getting on a different medication that is more effective. Your body may have become immune to your current inhaler or medication making it practically useless.

82. Concurrent health problems can contribute to your asthma symptoms. Many people with allergies find that their asthma symptoms become worse around allergy triggers. If you keep on top of your concurrent health problems, you'll be less likely to be triggered into an acute asthma attack. Ask your doctor if your other diagnoses could contribute to your struggle with asthma.

83. A great tip that can help you manage your asthma is to learn how to keep your stress levels in check. There are many variables that can trigger asthma and stress is one of them. Learning how to manage your stress will also help you manage your asthma.

84. Asthma can be triggered by cigarette smoke. People that have asthma are most often times very sensitive to it. You should take great steps

to make sure no one smokes in your car, in your home, or around you anywhere. This will help you immensely when you are trying to avoid asthma attacks, and stay healthy in general!

85. Let your friends know that they should not give you gifts of household plants. Plants can be a severe trigger for certain asthmatics. Having them constantly in your home would be like fighting a war with your environment every day. If someone does give you a plant, see if it can be planted outside. If it can't be moved outdoors, thank them nicely for the gift and then give it away later.

86. Beta 2 antagonists that can be inhaled are long term asthma control medicines that can be taken every day. They may also have risks for certain people as well. When you are taking these medications it is now recommended they be used along with corticosteroids that can be inhaled.

87. Keep in close contact with your allergist to let him know if your medication is working correctly to control your symptoms. Make him aware if your medication seems to be not working as well as it once may have. Your dosage or medication may need to be changed in order to help you.

88. You may want to get into a support group if you have asthma. The people in the group are in the same situation as you so they know what you have to go through everyday. Also, they may have personal tips of what you can do to control your asthma symptoms.

89. Use the right medication to control your asthma. Have you noticed that you can only prevent your asthma attack by using your inhaler more than twice a week? Do you have to refill your prescription several times a year? It might be a sign to visit your doctor and ask for a different medication to control your symptoms better.

90. Stop what you are doing when you feel that an asthma attack is coming. This is especially true when you are driving or operating heavy machinery. Explain to the people around you what is going on as they may become overly excited which in return can stress you out even more.

91. Have your home inspected at least once a year for mold and other spores. Many asthmatics, especially children, can have their asthma exacerbated by exposure to these allergens. Living in a home full of mold spores can even trigger repeated asthma attacks to the point of

permanently damaging a child's respiratory system.

92. Be cautious when taking medications with asthma. Even some over the counter drugs, such as non-steroidal anti-inflammatory medications, may worsen asthma symptoms. If you are taking an over-the-counter medicine, be alert to changes in your asthma symptoms or for indications of an asthma attack. It may be necessary to avoid certain medications, in order to keep your asthma under control.

93. Stay indoors during high pollen count days. Pollen and other airborne allergens account for many asthma symptoms. When pollen counts reach higher levels, the number of patients in the ER with severe asthma attacks increases. Avoid an attack, by staying indoors with an air conditioner or other air filtering system.

94. Focus on breathing through your nose to reduce the loss of excessive carbon dioxide, especially during strenuous activities. Breathing through your mouth can cause a sudden decrease in carbon dioxide levels, making your airways more prone to contraction. Breathing through your nose keeps levels more stable, making it easier to manage your asthma.

95. Wash your bedding, including your pillowcases, at least weekly, using hot water and chlorinated bleach. This will be more effective at killing dust mites than the use of liquid washing detergent alone. You have to wash bedding regularly to prevent the ones that do survive from continuing to multiply and causing problems.

96. Some over the counter decongestants can actually be used to help treat your asthma symptoms. This is because they work to break up the clutter that is in your lungs, allowing for a more open airway. Give them a try next time you have symptoms.

97. When suffering from asthma do not leave your care solely in your doctor's hands. Rather become a proactive member of a patient and doctor team. Learn as much as you can about yourself, your symptoms, and your care plan. And help your doctor design an even better plan such that asthma's interference in your life is minimal.

98. Know, and make sure your friends and your family know first aid for asthma attacks. This will ensure that in case of an emergency, the people around you are likely to know how to handle the

situation properly. Also, always remember to keep your relief inhaler with you at all times.

99. It is important that you do not get too stressed out if you suffer from asthma. Stress and panic are all major causes of asthma attacks. Also, try not lose your temper either. Getting angry can cause your breathing to become labored, which in turn, can trigger asthma attacks.

100.   Your doctor may thing that corticosteroids are the best relief from your asthma attacks. This is especially true if you have really bad attacks. They may be a little harder to diagnose but can be swallowed or injected in the case of an attack to open up your passages more effectively.

101.   Use natural remedies for your asthma. While doctor-prescribed medication might be necessary to prevent deadly attacks, a healthy diet will help to improve everyday life. Beta carotene's promote healthy mucus membranes in your mouth and nose which help to reduce the chances of serious asthma attacks.

102.   Keep your stress level as low as humanly possible. As anxiety levels increase due to everyday problems, so do asthma symptoms. If you experience wheezing and coughing several

times a day, consider stress relief techniques such as regular exercises and stretching and breathing exercises. Also, be sure you get enough sleep to deal with the stresses of everyday life.

103.   Try to reduce the amount of environmental allergens and pollutants, such as dust, pollens, pet hair, molds and fungi, and food particles. Keeping your house clean can make a huge difference for your asthma symptoms. Buying an air filter or purifier, or even cleaning out the filters in your AC system can also help.

104.   If you have children with asthma, complete a regular inspection of your home. The most common triggers of asthma attacks in children are dust, mold and other harmful spores in the air. Checking your home once a year for these air pollutants is an effective way to prevent and treat your child's asthma attacks.

105.   If you suffer from asthma and you have carpet in your home, you may want to consider getting rid of it and replacing it with hardwood floors. Carpets tend to collect dust and other unhealthy materials that can trigger asthma symptoms and attacks. If you do keep your carpet, be sure to vacuum it often.

106.   Change your sheets and comforter once a week, and wash them in hot water. One of the best ways to prevent attacks or common triggers is to ensure your home is clean and dry. Your bedding starts to collect dust, dander, dirt and other debris that can pollute the air you breathe. Frequent washing in hot water ensures these pollutants are kept to a minimum.

107.   If you suffer from asthma and do not smoke, make sure to avoid people who do smoke. Inhaling smoke from tobacco products can compromise your lung function, which then makes you more susceptible to an attack. The risk of an attack from cigarette smoke is increased as the space you are in decreases.

108.   Hay fever and colds can worsen asthma symptoms so prepare to need increased treatments. Treatment may be increased in these cases as many illnesses have side effects that can cause flare ups in your asthma. Your doctor may need to add new treatments to your typical asthma regimen until you are well.

109.   Join an online or offline support group. Extremely severe asthma can be debilitating and prevent one from living a full life. Others who suffer from asthma can give you immeasurable

amounts of support and advice, and help you keep up with new medical developments.

110. Engage your support network to help you manage your asthma. Talk to your friends and family about items that trigger attacks and enroll them in helping you make environmental or lifestyle changes to help you manage your asthma. The more knowledgeable your network is about your condition, the more easily they can support you.

111. Know what triggers your asthma and how to avoid them. Triggers are different for each person, so it may take some time to figure out what yours are. Keep a diary of them. Once you find out what your triggers are, try to avoid or limit your contact with them.

112. Take a friend or member of your family with you when you visit your doctor. Often, you are discussing so much information with your doctor that it can be difficult to keep track of all the data. Having someone with you gives you another set of ears to listen to the information and think of relevant questions. As a side benefit, having someone with you hear what the doctor says can help you engage your support network in your efforts to manage your asthma.

113.   Be aware of how your pets may affect your asthma. Ideally, an asthma sufferer should not have any fur bearing pet because of the pet dander shed by all furry animals, even those considered low allergen. At the same time, if you frequently visit friends with pets, take appropriate precautions to lessen the effects of exposure to dander during your visit.

114.   For temporary relief of asthma symptoms there are quick-relief medications. They are oral corticosteroids and bronchodilators. Bronchodilators are often called rescue medication and open up airways and allow more air to flow through. Corticosteroids are designed for short-term use and are either swallowed or given by injection. They work by treating inflammation in airways.

115.   If you struggle with asthma, be sure to keep in contact with your doctor. If the medications that you are taking are not as effective as they once were, contact your doctor immediately. Your doctor will be able to increase your dosage or recommend you to a better medication that will meet your asthma needs.

116.   If you suffer from asthma, you should not smoke or expose yourself to any type of vapors or fumes. This means avoidance of all tobacco products, as well as taking into consideration any smoke or vapors you might be exposed to in a prospective workplace.

117.   You should stay home as much as possible when it is humid outside or when there is a lot of pollen in the air. Humidity and pollen will make it hard for you to breathe. If you must go outside, you can wear a mask over your nose and mouth.

118.   A great tip that can help you get over an asthma attack is to try drinking a few cups of coffee. Coffee can help when you're having an asthma attack because the caffeine opens up the airways. With your airways opened, you'll be able to breathe much better.

119.   If you are going to exercise, start very slowly. Sudden exercise such as taking off running can trigger asthma for most people. You can exercise, but do some warming up exercises that will gradually increase your heart rate until you feel comfortable with harder exercises. Do not force yourself to exercise if you feel you are going to have an asthma attack.

120.   You may want to avoid getting pets, especially those with longer fur, if you have asthma. For many people, pet dander and fur is one of the major triggers of asthma attacks. If you really want to get a pet, try to get one with short fur or get an aquatic animal, like a fish.

121.   When you have asthma, you should always be under a doctors care. You will probably be prescribed medicine that should make it easier for you to breath. If you find that your medicine is not working well, you need to contact your doctor as soon as you can, and they can find a different drug that will help you.

122.   Leukotriene inhibitors are a very popular treatment for people that have asthma. This type of medication will work to stop chemical substances that can cause an asthma attack. It is very important that if you are prescribed these, you make sure to take it exactly how your doctor tells you to.

123.   When dealing with asthma, you should limit your contact with animals. Many people who have asthma also have an allergy to pets. Even if you do not have an allergy to pets, pets can carry trigger substances, such as dirt, in their fur.

These substances could cause an attack without you being allergic to pets.

124.   Leukotriene inhibitors can help control the symptoms of asthma. Leukotriene inhibitors work to prevent leukotrienes. Leukotriene are chemicals that may cause your lungs to get inflamed which can lead to an asthma attack. Leukotriene is an oral therapy for the treatment of asthma, but it is not as effective as inhaled corticosteroids.

125.   Raw apple cider vinegar is an excellent treatment for those who suffer from asthma. Mix two tablespoons with eight ounces of water or apple juice and drink up to three times daily. If you use water, honey can be added to make it more palatable. Look for raw apple cider vinegar in the health food section of most grocery stores.

126.   Be aware that your asthma medication may need to be adjusted if you are suffering from a cold, flu or hay fever. Some illnesses create issues that make it necessary to increase medication temporarily. Your doctor may need to add new treatments to your typical asthma regimen until you are well.

127.   If your doctor prescribes you a preventative inhaler, use it! Consider your preventative inhaler to be part of your daily pharmaceutical regimen, just like any other medication. If you don't use the inhaler, the medication it contains can't help you. Plus, if your doctor can't trust you to take your medications, they can't effectively treat your asthma.

128.   Keep an asthma diary to help you identify substances that trigger attacks or worsen symptoms. In this diary, keep track of foods and activities to help you pinpoint those items that cause asthma attacks. Your asthma diary is also beneficial when working with your doctor on your long-term management plan.

129.   When traveling and staying in hotel rooms with a severe asthmatic, be sure to explain the situation to the hotel staff in advance. You need a room that is not only non-smoking but that has never been smoked in, and you also need a non-smoking floor. If the hotel can't accomodate that request, find a different one.

130.   Smoke should always be avoided when you suffer from asthma. Smoke and chemicals have been known to trigger asthma attacks. You should stay far away from smoke of any kind,

chemicals and vapors. These environmental conditions can exacerbate your asthma symptoms. If someone smokes around you, ask them politely if they could smoke when you are not around.

131.   Control or eliminate cockroaches. On top of being a general health hazard, cockroaches produce dander that can trigger asthma and allergy symptoms. If you do have roaches, use Boric acid or traps to kill them instead of chemical pesticides. These can irritate your bronchial pathways and trigger an attack too.

132.   Learn all that you can learn about the condition you have. Education is a priceless tool in finding the proper treatment for your asthma. Keep current with treatments and ensure you have the greatest possible care that you can have. The best way to ensure this is to know as much as you can about asthma and your options for treatment.

133.   You should stay home as much as possible when it is humid outside or when there is a lot of pollen in the air. Humidity and pollen will make it hard for you to breathe. If you must go outside, you can wear a mask over your nose and mouth.

134.   Buy cleaning products that are labeled as environmentally-friendly. This will not cost you more, and they are just as efficient as chemical products. These green products will reduce the risk of asthma attacks and allow you to keep your house clean at the same time. Look for non-toxic cleaning products.

135.   If you're caught without your inhaler when you have an attack, grab a cup of coffee. The caffeine in the beverage will open up your airways and allow you to breathe a little easier. If you don't have a caffeinated beverage on hand, the small amounts of caffeine in a chocolate bar can also help.

136.   A healthy diet can help you to better manage your asthma. Studies have shown that processed foods, sugar, and trans fats can bring about inflammation which can trigger asthma. You don't have to cut these foods out entirely, but you should keep them to a minimum.

137.   When you have asthma, it is vital that you avoid cleaning products. Many chemicals contained in common cleaning products can aggravate your asthma, triggering an attack. If

you clean the home, there are many natural products that are safe to use.

138.   Asthma can be triggered by cigarette smoke. People that have asthma are most often times very sensitive to it. You should take great steps to make sure no one smokes in your car, in your home, or around you anywhere. This will help you immensely when you are trying to avoid asthma attacks, and stay healthy in general!

139.   There is help for when you feel an asthma attack coming on and your inhaler is not with you. Caffeinated drinks can help you as they open your airways. Drink a couple of cups of coffee, tea, or hot chocolate before the full onset of your attack to minimize its negative effects.

140.   Talk to a social worker if you have asthma and no health insurance. You will need asthma medications, and if you are unable to afford them, a social worker can find a hospital or clinic that can offer you medication for free or for a little cost.

141.   If money is a factor in taking your medications properly, or even at all, ask your doctor for alternatives. They may be able to prescribe a lower cost medication, one with

coupon offers or discounts, as well as provide you with free samples from the pharmaceutical companies. Their goal is to keep you out of the hospital.

142.   Keep track of upcoming weather conditions that may affect your asthma. Some sufferers are affected more strongly than others by changes in barometric pressure or humidity. If you are one of these, being aware of upcoming storms or changes in weather to help you find ways to manage the changes in weather to limit the impact on your asthma symptoms.

143.   If you are prone to attacks during allergy season, make use of over the counter allergy medications. While allergies and asthma are not the same, they do have many of the same mechanisms, and many people have both seasonal allergies and asthma. A seasonal allergy attack can compound the effects of asthma.

144.   For asthma sufferers having contact with pets or other animals need to be minimized. While allergies to dander or animal hair can possibly complicate your asthma, even those with no such allergies can have asthma attacks by inhaling the pollen and dust animals usually carry about with them.

145.   If you have asthma, you are especially sensitive to things you breathe into your lungs. It is important to avoid whatever triggers your asthma. In some people, this will be cigarette smoke. For others, it is chemical fumes or other vapors that can irritate the lungs and bring on an attack.

146.   When dealing with an asthma attack, it is important to stay calm. Wait thirty seconds to try your inhaler after using it the first time. If the attack gets worse doesn't get better, then get help immediately. Have some one call for an ambulance or take you to the hospital. Breathe into a paper bag, which will reduce your breathing rate during the trip.

147.   Try to keep yourself at optimum health for the best asthma management. Make sure you drink plenty of water, get plenty of sleep and exercise regularly. This will keep your body and immune system strong and lessen the chance of a severe asthma attack and a trip to the emergency room.

148.   Somehow, an asthma attack seems to get worse the harder you try to breathe. Here are some tips to alleviate the discomfort of an

ordinary attack. When you begin to have symptoms, breathe through your nose, try to relax and don't fight your breathing. Finally, try to reduce your breathing rate to how it felt before the attack started.

149.   Reduce the symptoms of asthma by removing carpets from your home, which can hold in all sorts of environmental hazards that can trigger a severe asthma attack, especially if you have pets. Furthermore, if you have a cat or dog, do not let them in your room. You breathe very deeply in your sleep, so the bedroom is the worst place for fur, dust or dander.

150.   Avoid keeping potted plants in your home. Certain plants might have a smell or change the nature of the air you breathe in a way that triggers asthma. If you want to keep plants, pay close attention to your symptoms and be ready to remove the plants if you notice any changes.

151.   You do not have to be physically inactive just because you have asthma. Unlike decades ago, when asthma treatments were few and far between, there are plenty of different asthma inhalers and medications that you can take prior to and after performing physical activities. Ask

your doctor for the best treatment for your specific needs.

152.   Get the flu vaccine every year if you suffer from asthma. Respiratory or sinus issues that can come from a bout with the flu can really do a number on an asthma sufferer. Taking the preventive tack of getting the vaccine can save you some serious suffering down the road.

153.   If you or your children are struggling with asthma, it is important to have your home inspected yearly for asthma triggers. Triggers for asthma in the home are dust, mold, and any other spores that may be present in your home. These triggers will often affect children more than adults.

154.   Have your home inspected at least once a year for mold and mildew if you have asthma. As bad as mold and mildew is for healthy people, it is even worse for people with asthma because it can decrease lung function and make breathing harder. If you suspect you do have mold in your home, be sure to let your doctor know.

155.   Use a peak flow meter regularly. A peak flow meter measures how much air your lungs can put out. If you keep track of your peak flow, you can

notice changes in your airflow capacity before you even start to notice symptoms of an attack, and take preventative action to stop it.

156.   A doctor will generally prescribe two different asthma inhalers. One of them will be a brown inhaler which should be taken regularly, and the other will be a blue inhaler for emergencies. You should always carry your blue inhaler with you in case you have an asthma attack, and make sure to stay on top of refilling the prescription as needed. In the event of an asthma attack, if the blue inhaler is not helping, do not hesitate to call 911.

157.   When you are trying to prevent asthma, you should avoid smoke. Smoke can cause asthma attacks. The fumes from chemicals, or smoke from cigarettes, should be avoided at all costs. Exposing yourself to these pollutants can have a significant effect on your asthma symptoms. If you live with or near a smoker, find a way to politely ask that they not smoke around you or your living spaces.

158.   Wear sunglasses in the spring and summer. Many people with asthma suffer from seasonal allergies as well, or are at least sensitive to pollen. Wearing sunglasses keeps pollen and dust out of

your eyes, which can reduce symptoms of allergies. A runny nose or other allergy symptom can easily trigger an asthma attack.

159. If riding in a car with an asthmatic, make sure the air conditioner or heater is set to "recirculate". This setting uses the same air that's already in the car to cycle through the heating or cooling system. Other settings will allow air from outside the car to enter, and this outside air can contain pollen, pollution, or other irritants.

160. One potential solution to your asthma problem might be a leukotriene inhibitor. Leukotrienes are chemical compounds that tend to aggravate asthma symptoms and bring on attacks. They can cause the muscles of the throat to constrict involuntarily. Consult a physician about your particular case and the potential suitability of a leukotriene-inhibiting treatment.

161. Do not use a vaporizer or humidifier unless you are sure it's been thoroughly cleaned. If it is not clean you end up getting bacteria growth in the damp interior of the machine, and that ends up flooding the air you want to humidify with allergens.

162.   Take care of your body from the inside out to avoid getting sick. When you get sick, you will have a lot of trouble breathing, which can exacerbate your asthma symptoms. In the morning, consume various fruits that contain a high dose of vitamin C to prevent from getting colds.

163.   Try to keep yourself at optimum health for the best asthma management. Make sure you drink plenty of water, get plenty of sleep and exercise regularly. This will keep your body and immune system strong and lessen the chance of a severe asthma attack and a trip to the emergency room.

164.   Sometimes you can be having an asthma attack and not know it. This is normally called a silent asthma attack. A way to tell if you are having a silent asthma attack is to make sure that your fingernails or lips are not purple, as this indicates a lack of oxygen to your lungs.

165.   Be careful of taking common medications if you have asthma. Many can trigger an asthma attack. Among these are things like aspirin, beta-blockers, ibuprofen, various migraine medications, cold medications and more. Always consult with your doctor before taking any over-

the-counter medication. In fact, you should see your doctor about any medical questions to be sure you are taking proper care of yourself.

166.   Think about getting a flu shot. If you have asthma regularly, your lungs have more risks have getting infected. A flu shot should protect your lungs from common types of infections. If you have a child with asthma, you should definitely get them a flu shot to prevent them from developing any severe lung infections.

167.   When dealing with asthma, you should limit your contact with animals. Many people who have asthma also have an allergy to pets. Even if you do not have an allergy to pets, pets can carry trigger substances, such as dirt, in their fur. These substances could cause an attack without you being allergic to pets.

168.   If you suffer from asthma, you might want to check if you have any allergies to certain foods or your environment. There are many things that could contribute such as pets, cleaning products, feather pillows or bed, even certain perfumes. Dairy products as well as refined foods like white flour and sugar likely causes.

169.   Cover padded or fabric covered items such as mattresses in allergen-proof covers to lessen the amount of dust and allergens captured in these items. Since fabric covered items easily collect allergens, not covering them can cause a significant increase in asthma symptoms or attacks. Keeping these items encased in allergen-proof covers can lessen asthma symptoms.

170.   Use a peak flow meter regularly. A peak flow meter measures how much air your lungs can put out. If you keep track of your peak flow, you can notice changes in your airflow capacity before you even start to notice symptoms of an attack, and take preventative action to stop it.

171.   For temporary relief of asthma symptoms there are quick-relief medications. They are oral corticosteroids and bronchodilators. Bronchodilators are often called rescue medication and open up airways and allow more air to flow through. Corticosteroids are designed for short-term use and are either swallowed or given by injection. They work by treating inflammation in airways.

172.   Talk with your doctor and determine if supplements could help you manage your Asthma. Natural supplements such as Licorice

Root, Marshmallow Root, Gingko Biloba and Mullein help some Asthma sufferers control their symptoms. You may find adding one or more of these supplements to your diet helps you manage your condition, but be sure to discuss with your doctor before beginning one.

173.	A doctor will generally prescribe two different asthma inhalers. One of them will be a brown inhaler which should be taken regularly, and the other will be a blue inhaler for emergencies. You should always carry your blue inhaler with you in case you have an asthma attack, and make sure to stay on top of refilling the prescription as needed. In the event of an asthma attack, if the blue inhaler is not helping, do not hesitate to call 911.

174.	Add onions to your daily diet. Onions contain a chemical called diphenyl-thiosulfate, which has been shown to have anti-inflammatory and anti-asthmatic effects. Eating more onions can reduce your need for pharmaceutical interventions in order to treat your asthma symptoms, by increasing your body's natural ability to reduce inflammation in your lungs.

175.	A dehumidifier can help ease your asthma symptoms. The wettest season is typically the season when you experience the worst asthma aggravation. A dehumidifier can make your home a pleasant refuge from seasonal asthma triggers. Dry air is easier for the asthma sufferer to breathe. You should always ensure that the dehumidifier you use - like all air-treatment devices - is clean before using it.

176.   Smoke is one of the worst asthma aggravators. It goes without saying that asthma sufferers should not smoke, but some consideration on the part of those they live with is called for, too. A household that includes an asthma sufferer must be a smoke-free one. Smokers in the household must be willing to keep the indoor air clean out of medical necessity.

177.   Any time that pollen counts go up, anyone suffering from asthma would be wise to keep their outdoors time to a minimum. Asthma symptoms are not the same as allergic reactions, but allergies and asthma attacks have many common triggers. The air quality information should be used to find out when it is better to stay indoors to avoid irritants present in the air.

178.   If you have problems with asthma, consider using plastic covers on your pillows and

mattress. These bedding materials are extremely porous and provide a fertile harbor for dust, mold, pollen and other irritants that can bring on an asthma attack. Sheathing them in plastic - especially if you do it immediately after purchase - can keep your pillows and mattresses from turning into asthma traps.

179.   If you suffer from asthma, always make sure that you breathe through your nose during any type of vigorous activity. If you have to open your mouth to breath and find yourself losing control, just stop, calm yourself, focus on normalizing your breathing methods and then go back to doing your activity.

180.   If repainting a room is in your future, purchase a quality mask first to protect your lungs from paint fumes. Not surprisingly, paint fumes are a known irritant for asthma. Specially designed masks can filter out these fumes. Refrain from using any substance or chemical that aggravate your asthma.

181.   You should avoid smoking at all costs and being exposed to vapors and perfumes if you suffer from asthma. This means you should stay away from all tobacco products and carefully consider the jobs you apply to, especially in

factories, as you may be exposed to harmful smoke or vapors.

182.   Avoid living with smokers. Ask your partner to quit if you have asthma. If you absolutely have to live with smokers, try to get them to smoke outside the house. In the worst case scenario, buy some smoke-eating candles and air out your house as much as possible so that no harmful chemicals remain in the air.

183.   A great tip that can help your child deal with asthma is to inform as many people as possible about your child's condition. You should tell their teacher, the babysitter, and everyone else that has the responsibility of looking after your child. They'll understand your child's needs and they'll be able to help.

184.   To prevent sudden attacks work to learn your triggers. After you have an attack, make a note about the environment you were in. In time you should begin to see patterns and be prepared for environmental factors that may cause issues for you. This will help limit the effect your asthma has on your day to day life.

185.   If you have asthma, and you have no choice but to live in a cold environment, try not to

spend too much outside when it is cold. The cold will worsen your asthma symptoms or cause attacks. Spend as much time as you can in a hot environment and when you have to go outside, wear a scarf.

186.   Be wary of what pain relievers you use. People with asthma try not to use aspirin and NAIDs, or Non-Steroidal Anti-Inflammatory Drugs, like Advil, Motrin, and Aleve, because there is a possibility of them worsening your asthma symptoms. Instead, try to use acetaminophen, more commonly known as Tylenol, to help relieve your pain.

187.   If you have children with asthma, complete a regular inspection of your home. The most common triggers of asthma attacks in children are dust, mold and other harmful spores in the air. Checking your home once a year for these air pollutants is an effective way to prevent and treat your child's asthma attacks.

188.   To alleviate or prevent asthma attacks, minimize how often and much you come into contact with animals. Even if you are not allergic to pet hair or dander, a common occurrence with asthma, you can have an attack triggered by the dirt or pet dander simply being in the air. If you

have pets in the home, vacuum often to limit pet-triggered air pollutants.

189.   Avoid bringing plants into your home. Unfortunately, this includes decorative bouquets and similar gifts. The pollen and scents produced by these plants can trigger asthma symptoms, or they can trigger the environmental allergies that go along with asthma for many sufferers. If someone does bring flowers into your home, thank them politely but remove the flowers at the first sign of symptoms.

190.   If you have children with asthma, be aware of their symptoms and watch for them. Many children do not want to report symptoms because they are afraid of being removed from a fun activity. If you notice a child suffering from symptoms, gently encourage use of an inhaler without insisting that they be removed from the situation.

191.   Shower or bathe each evening before going to bed to remove any allergens that can trigger an asthma attack. Sleeping with allergens on your skin or hair can not only cause an attack, but may make you even more sensitive to specific triggers over time.

192.   When traveling and staying in hotel rooms with a severe asthmatic, be sure to explain the situation to the hotel staff in advance. You need a room that is not only non-smoking but that has never been smoked in, and you also need a non-smoking floor. If the hotel can't accomodate that request, find a different one.

193.   Do your research. While you should always follow your doctor's orders, do not rely on them as your sole source of information. Check out or buy books on asthma and look into support forums online. Not only will you be sure to see many options for care, you doctor will appreciate having a well-informed patient.

194.   In order to combat asthma, you may need to get rid of your houseplants. Some indoor plants produce pollen and other irritants that can aggravate asthma. Even plants that do not make their own allergens contribute to your asthma troubles by harboring dust and dirt. Eliminating houseplants can make a small but definitely positive impact on your asthma condition.

195.   Any allergy can have a deleterious synergy with an asthma condition, and food allergies are no different. If you have asthma problems, a clinical food allergy test can help you pinpoint

problem foods. A mild food allergy could exacerbate your asthma without your noticing. A full medical test can help you identify foods you need to avoid to keep your asthma in check.

196.   You may need to make some lifestyle changes, especially if you develop asthma as an adult. If you are overweight or out of shape, do some light exercise every day and quit smoking, if you are a smoker. These changes may be difficult, but will lead to better health in the long run, and less problems with asthma.

197.   An ounce of prevention goes a long way in battling asthma. Asthma is a defense mechanism in your body, make sure that your body doesn't trigger this process so you can avoid acute asthma attacks. Your doctor can help you determine which maintenance medicines will be best for your type of asthma.

198.   You do not have to be physically inactive just because you have asthma. Unlike decades ago, when asthma treatments were few and far between, there are plenty of different asthma inhalers and medications that you can take prior to and after performing physical activities. Ask your doctor for the best treatment for your specific needs.

199.   There are two types of asthma medications that are used by people in their on going hunt for relief from their condition. One is a long term management medication and the other is one to control an asthma attack. Your doctor may recommend one or a combination of both of them.

200.   Buy a dehumidifier if you suffer from seasonal allergies. Dry environments are much better for asthmatics than high humidity areas. The use of a dehumidifier will create the best home for your asthma issues. Doing so will help out the entire family as well since the house will be more pleasant to live in.

201.   If you have asthma, know your triggers. What is it that causes an asthma attack to come on? Many common triggers are allergies and irritants. For some, it is exercise or extreme temperatures. Emotional or anxiety issues can also cause asthma type attacks. Knowing what causes your attack can also be what will help you find a proper treatment.

202.   If you have been diagnosed with asthma then you want to be sure that your doctor prescribes for you a rescue inhaler. You will want

to bring this rescue inhaler with you wherever you go. The reason for this is very simple: you simply never know when you will have an asthma attack.

203.   For asthma patients who are purchasing new furniture, try to make sure that you keep your windows open for a few days when you get your furniture so that it can air out. Many people who suffer from asthma find that the smells of new furniture make their asthma symptoms much worse.

204.   An increased propensity for asthma attacks has been linked with the utilization of multiple cleaning products. The more you use, the greater the risk of an attack. Use organic cleaning products since they don't have irritating chemicals.

205.   A yearly home inspection by a qualified professional for common asthma triggers, such as mold spores and dust, is a must for asthma sufferers. Removing any of these substance's if they are present in your home can reduce the number of asthma attacks suffered and make life more comfortable for the entire family.

206.   Join a support group, online or in "real life", to find help from your peers. Asthma, especially severe asthma, can be a debilitating condition and prevent you from participating fully in daily life. Others who suffer from asthma can give you immeasurable amounts of support and advice, and help you keep up with new medical developments.

207.   If you suffer from asthma, you should be aware that animals can be a trigger for asthma attacks. While you might not have any specific animal related allergies, animals do accumulate dirt and other harmful substances that can trigger an attack when you go near them. In particular, you should be careful around common pets like dogs and cats.

208.   To decrease your asthma symptoms, you should try to avoid going outside during humid seasons. You should also try to stay inside when the seasons are changing. The amount of pollen in the air increases with a season change. Pollen is one of the main triggers for asthma attacks and other asthma symptoms.

209.   One of the most common things people do to make their asthma condition worse is putting their hands near their face. Your hands touch

many different things throughout the day and when they are dirty, the particles can transfer from your hands to your face and then ultimately to your lungs. In order to prevent further complicating your asthma condition and reduce the chance of an asthma attack, wash your hands frequently and keep them away from your face.

210.   If you have asthma troubles, make sure that you get a flu vaccination every year. Although this has no direct effect on your asthma, preventing the flu is in your best interests. Respiratory infections are more aggravating, more debilitating and harder to shake for asthma sufferers. Staying free of the flu can save you a lot of hassle.

211.   Clean your house and get rid of clutter. Asthma attacks are often triggered by the presence of dust in the air. Cluttered surfaces are harder to dust than clear ones, and hard floors are better than carpeting or rugs. Dust with a damp cloth to avoid throwing it up into the air.

212.   Knowing the correct way to use an inhaler is essential. When you spray the inhaler into your mouth, you cannot just lightly inhale. When you spray the inhaler, be sure to breathe in as deeply as you can for two to three seconds. Holding it

in will allow the medicine to open up your bronchial passages and relieve your attack.

213.   Be careful of taking common medications if you have asthma. Many can trigger an asthma attack. Among these are things like aspirin, beta-blockers, ibuprofen, various migraine medications, cold medications and more. Always consult with your doctor before taking any over-the-counter medication. In fact, you should see your doctor about any medical questions to be sure you are taking proper care of yourself.

214.   Wash your bedding regularly, at least once a week. Your bedding might contain dust and microscopic acarids which can cause asthma. You should also place a protective plastic cover on your mattress since you cannot wash it. Keep your clean bedding in a drawer where it will not get dusty.

215.   Avoid being in contact with pets. Pets carry a lot of dust and other impurities on them. If you have a pet, wash it every week, and try keeping its hairs as short as possible. If you are going to be in contact with an animal, perhaps you should wear a mask.

216.   Clean up your house from food and water. Keep your food inside the fridge. When you let food or water sit, you are attracting small bugs and roaches, which can trigger allergic reactions. If you need to keep food outside of your fridge, consider getting a food pantry or opening your windows.

217.   If you are going to exercise, start very slowly. Sudden exercise such as taking off running can trigger asthma for most people. You can exercise, but do some warming up exercises that will gradually increase your heart rate until you feel comfortable with harder exercises. Do not force yourself to exercise if you feel you are going to have an asthma attack.

218.   Medications can be taken on a regular basis to control inflammation in your airways. Inhaled corticosteroids such as cromolyn and leukotriene modifiers are some such medications. Consult with your doctor about which one is the best for you. You may need to try several of them.

219.   There is help for when you feel an asthma attack coming on and your inhaler is not with you. Caffeinated drinks can help you as they open your airways. Drink a couple of cups of

coffee, tea, or hot chocolate before the full onset of your attack to minimize its negative effects.

220.   If you have asthma, know your triggers. What is it that causes an asthma attack to come on? Many common triggers are allergies and irritants. For some, it is exercise or extreme temperatures. Emotional or anxiety issues can also cause asthma type attacks. Knowing what causes your attack can also be what will help you find a proper treatment.

221.   IF you have asthma, you should consider buying a dehumidifier. Though you may not be aware of it, high levels of humidity in indoor spaces can increase dust mites, which then can affect asthma. A dehumidifying device reduces the moisture in the air.

222.   Keeping yourself healthy can be a way to control your asthma better. The common cold, as well as viruses and bacterial infections can cause a flare up or attack of your asthma. Especially colds which produce mucus or a nasal drip that can end up in your lungs.

223.   Make sure to take all of your asthma medications exactly as your doctor prescribes them, even if you haven't been suffering any

symptoms lately. Not having symptoms doesn't mean your asthma went away; it just means your medications are working! This includes your preventative medications as well as your rescue inhaler.

224.   Household plants and flowers can act as an asthma attack trigger. The reason for this is that many of them carry pollen and other particles that can get into the air. They can cause problems even if the air is well circulated in the home. To be completely safe, don't bring plants and flowers into the home, and if someone has them delivered to your home, throw them out immediately.

225.   Try using a inhaler that prevents asthma every day, but you should know that one of the side effects is mouth infections of teeth and gums. Prevent these unnecessary side effects by gargling and brushing your teeth right after you use the inhaler.

226.   Get in the habit of sleeping on your side or stomach to improve your quality of sleep and absorption of oxygen during sleep. Sleeping on your back increases the likelihood you breathe through your mouth, which can worsen asthma symptoms. By sleeping on your side or stomach,

your body naturally breathes more shallowly through your nose, making it easier for your lungs to work efficiently.

227.   Asthma sufferers should have minimal contact with animals including pets. While an allergy to animal hair or dander is a possible asthma complication, even those sufferers free of such allergies can experience an asthma attack caused by the dust and pollen all animals tend to carry along with them.

228.   Asthma sufferers should definitely stay indoors more when pollen increases. While asthma isn't an allergy, many allergy irritants can affect it. Many areas provide air quality information publicly, allowing you to stay indoors when the air outside is poor.

229.   Include more vitamin B6 foods in your diet. Research has shown that pyridoxine, commonly referred to as vitamin B6, can lower the number of asthma events and lessen their intensity. Pyridoxine (vitamin B6) is instrumental in the production of specific molecules which help the bronchial tissue to relax. A banana is a great food that is rich in vitamin B6.

230.   Getting thinner and more active will actually improve your asthma. Being heavier set and sedentary can be agitators to breathing. It can be difficult to start at first, but it does get better. Try something easy at first, such as water exercises or cycling on a stationary bike. The more you get closer to a healthy BMI, the less stress you will cause yourself when you are breathing.

231.   Asthma can be a scary thing. Your airways tighten up and breathing becomes increasingly difficult. For someone without this disease, it is hard to understand the importance of being in control and having the proper treatments available to you. As you read on you will see some great ideas on how you can better manage your asthma.

232.   You should stay home as much as possible when it is humid outside or when there is a lot of pollen in the air. Humidity and pollen will make it hard for you to breathe. If you must go outside, you can wear a mask over your nose and mouth.

233.   Get a bronchodilator or an inhaler. These products usually allow you to breathe better a few seconds after you use them. There are risks inherent to using these products, but if you use

them as prescribed they should make your life easier. Ask your doctor about what kind of inhaler you should use.

234.   If you're using your inhaler more than twice a week, you should talk to your doctor about additional asthma treatments. An inhaler is meant only for emergency relief and if you're periodically relying on it, then your current asthma treatment isn't effective enough. Overuse of an inhaler can be harmful and you should avoid potential problems, right away.

235.   If you or your children are struggling with asthma, it is important to have your home inspected yearly for asthma triggers. Triggers for asthma in the home are dust, mold, and any other spores that may be present in your home. These triggers will often affect children more than adults.

236.   Stop what you are doing when you feel that an asthma attack is coming. This is especially true when you are driving or operating heavy machinery. Explain to the people around you what is going on as they may become overly excited which in return can stress you out even more.

237.   Asthma can range from a small annoyance to an all-out, life-threatening condition. To help prevent Asthma attacks, keep moderation in mind, especially when engaging in outdoor activities in hot weather. Hot and humid air can make breathing difficult for anyone, but for someone with Asthma, it can be deadly. If you have work to do outside, try and choose to do so early in the morning or late in the day and avoid the mid-day sun and heat.

238.   Be cautious when taking medications with asthma. Even some over the counter drugs, such as non-steroidal anti-inflammatory medications, may worsen asthma symptoms. If you are taking an over-the-counter medicine, be alert to changes in your asthma symptoms or for indications of an asthma attack. It may be necessary to avoid certain medications, in order to keep your asthma under control.

239.   Household plants and flowers can act as an asthma attack trigger. The reason for this is that many of them carry pollen and other particles that can get into the air. They can cause problems even if the air is well circulated in the home. To be completely safe, don't bring plants and flowers into the home, and if someone has

them delivered to your home, throw them out immediately.

240.   Know what triggers your asthma and how to avoid them. Triggers are different for each person, so it may take some time to figure out what yours are. Keep a diary of them. Once you find out what your triggers are, try to avoid or limit your contact with them.

241.   Be aware of how your pets may affect your asthma. Ideally, an asthma sufferer should not have any fur bearing pet because of the pet dander shed by all furry animals, even those considered low allergen. At the same time, if you frequently visit friends with pets, take appropriate precautions to lessen the effects of exposure to dander during your visit.

242.   Focus on breathing through your nose to reduce the loss of excessive carbon dioxide, especially during strenuous activities. Breathing through your mouth can cause a sudden decrease in carbon dioxide levels, making your airways more prone to contraction. Breathing through your nose keeps levels more stable, making it easier to manage your asthma.

243.   Wash your bedding, including your pillowcases, at least weekly, using hot water and chlorinated bleach. This will be more effective at killing dust mites than the use of liquid washing detergent alone. You have to wash bedding regularly to prevent the ones that do survive from continuing to multiply and causing problems.

244.   Educate yourself about asthma. The greater your knowledge base regarding asthma, the more involved you can be in determining treatment plans. Keep current with recent developments in asthma treatment and research so that you can maintain cutting edge care in your personal case. The only way for you gain this knowledge would be to learn what your type of condition is and the treatment options.

245.   It is important to avoid locations that have very cold air. Cold air is very hard to take in, and can leave you gasping at times. Thus, if you have asthma, make sure that this is taken into consideration when you are planning vacations or trips with friends and family.

246.   Every single week, get in the habit of washing your bed sheets. During the course of the day, dust mites will reside on your bed, which

can incite symptoms of asthma when you sleep. Clean your sheets to eliminate this dust mites and create a hygienic area for resting.

247.   Asthma can be triggered by environmental factors such as allergens, or it could be genetic. If asthma has occurred in your family, be aware of any symptoms of asthma you or your children may exhibit. Things in the environment like smoke, mold, dust and pollution can aggravate asthma. It is important to keep your family and self away from these things.

248.   Do not sweep your house when you clean it. This will send dust flying everywhere and make it hard for you to breathe. Instead, you should use a wet mop so that the dust and impurities stick to the floor. Avoid using aerosols while cleaning, as these products could trigger asthma.

249.   If you are out of shape, a solid exercise regimen can help improve your asthma symptoms. The fact is that under-exerting ourselves can lead the body to exhaustion more easily. By pushing your boundaries, you tone functions vital to your body's general balance, making your body less likely to go haywire.

250. A great tip that can help you manage your asthma is to learn how to keep your stress levels in check. There are many variables that can trigger asthma and stress is one of them. Learning how to manage your stress will also help you manage your asthma.

251. A great tip that can help you manage your asthma is to start using nutritional supplements. Supplements such as vitamin C, D, and B are all wonderful for preventing asthma. If you aren't getting enough vitamins from your food you should definitely look into purchasing some of these vitamin supplements.

252. Be careful of what profession you choose if you have asthma. Certain jobs like painters, bakers, health workers, and farm workers involve using chemicals or materials that could worsen your asthma or cause an asthma attack. Try to stick with jobs in which you will be in a healthy environment all day.

253. Let your friends know that they should not give you gifts of household plants. Plants can be a severe trigger for certain asthmatics. Having them constantly in your home would be like fighting a war with your environment every day. If someone does give you a plant, see if it can be

planted outside. If it can't be moved outdoors, thank them nicely for the gift and then give it away later.

254.   Have your home inspected at least once a year for mold and other spores. Many asthmatics, especially children, can have their asthma exacerbated by exposure to these allergens. Living in a home full of mold spores can even trigger repeated asthma attacks to the point of permanently damaging a child's respiratory system.

255.   If your doctor prescribes you a preventative inhaler, use it! Consider your preventative inhaler to be part of your daily pharmaceutical regimen, just like any other medication. If you don't use the inhaler, the medication it contains can't help you. Plus, if your doctor can't trust you to take your medications, they can't effectively treat your asthma.

256.   If you are an asthma patient, be sure that you are drinking water that has been filtered. Unfiltered water could possibly contain allergens which could cause a severe asthma attack or flare up your symptoms. If you can afford it, you may want to consider only drinking water that has come from a bottle.

257.   Emotional issues, high stress and anxiety can also cause asthma symptoms. These may be treated with medications and or therapy, as well as eating properly, getting a good amount of exercise and making sure that you are getting a good eight hours of sleep or more, each and every night.

258.   Is it time for a new asthma medication? It is possible you need to try a new medication if you need to use your quick-relief inhaler anymore than twice a week. Also, if you need to refill your inhaler more than twice a year, or you wake up at night with asthma symptoms more than twice a week you also need to look into a change.

259.   If you are going on a plane trip with asthma medications, make sure to bring your written prescription along with you. The written prescription will help you get through security without difficulty, because it establishes that your nebulizer and supplies are medically necessary.

260.   Talk with your doctor and determine if supplements could help you manage your Asthma. Natural supplements such as Licorice Root, Marshmallow Root, Gingko Biloba and Mullein help some Asthma sufferers control

their symptoms. You may find adding one or more of these supplements to your diet helps you manage your condition, but be sure to discuss with your doctor before beginning one.

261.   If you struggle with asthma, be sure to keep in contact with your doctor. If the medications that you are taking are not as effective as they once were, contact your doctor immediately. Your doctor will be able to increase your dosage or recommend you to a better medication that will meet your asthma needs.

262.   If you find yourself without an inhaler when an asthma attack is coming on, try having a cold soda. The caffeine can actually open your airways and control the asthma. Preferably keep your inhaler on you at all times, but in case you find yourself without one, try drinking a caffeinated beverage.

263.   If you suffer from asthma, always make sure that you breathe through your nose during any type of vigorous activity. If you have to open your mouth to breath and find yourself losing control, just stop, calm yourself, focus on normalizing your breathing methods and then go back to doing your activity.

264.   If you are experiencing an asthma attack then you should sit down, lean forward, and put a warm compress on your chest to help relax those muscles. of course, while doing this use your rescue inhaler, or a plastic bag to help control your breathing. This should help get you through the attack without harm to your health.

265.   Concurrent health problems can contribute to your asthma symptoms. Many people with allergies find that their asthma symptoms become worse around allergy triggers. If you keep on top of your concurrent health problems, you'll be less likely to be triggered into an acute asthma attack. Ask your doctor if your other diagnoses could contribute to your struggle with asthma.

266.   You should use the AC as much as possible so that you can breathe fresh air. But make sure you clean up your AC unit regularly. If you are going to use a humidifier, clean it too. An unclean AC system could make your life absolutely miserable if you have asthma.

267.   If you enjoy using a vaporizer or a humidifier, you have to make sure it is clean before each use. These types of machines can build up a lot of dust and calcium, that you do

not want getting into the air you breath. You need to be breathing the cleanest air possible, at all times.

268.   Keeping your allergies in check is important in order to keep your asthma in check. Allergies and asthma commonly go together, and when your allergies or flairing up, your asthma probably will to. In addition to your inhaler, be sure to use an allergy medication when allergy season is at its peak.

269.   Avoid being around smoke and fumes. Smoke, including cigarette smoke and vehicle exhaust, contain small particles of dust and chemicals, which can irritate the bronchial linings. This irritation is dangerous for asthmatics, as it can interfere with breathing in an already compromised system. Breathing in cigarette smoke especially can trigger an asthma attack.

270.   Do not let having asthma get to you. Many people get depressed when they find out that they have asthma because they think their whole life will change. This is not true. As long as you take your treatments as directed by your doctor, you can continue to do most of the things that you used to.

271.   A yearly home inspection by a qualified professional for common asthma triggers, such as mold spores and dust, is a must for asthma sufferers. Removing any of these substance's if they are present in your home can reduce the number of asthma attacks suffered and make life more comfortable for the entire family.

272.   If money is a factor in taking your medications properly, or even at all, ask your doctor for alternatives. They may be able to prescribe a lower cost medication, one with coupon offers or discounts, as well as provide you with free samples from the pharmaceutical companies. Their goal is to keep you out of the hospital.

273.   When traveling and staying in hotel rooms with a severe asthmatic, be sure to explain the situation to the hotel staff in advance. You need a room that is not only non-smoking but that has never been smoked in, and you also need a non-smoking floor. If the hotel can't accomodate that request, find a different one.

274.   Get in the habit of sleeping on your side or stomach to improve your quality of sleep and absorption of oxygen during sleep. Sleeping on

your back increases the likelihood you breathe through your mouth, which can worsen asthma symptoms. By sleeping on your side or stomach, your body naturally breathes more shallowly through your nose, making it easier for your lungs to work efficiently.

275.   When you clean your home, as you should do regularly to minimize asthma symptoms, use all-natural cleaning products. Harsh chemical cleaners can give off fumes that may irritate your lungs and make your asthma symptoms worse. Many chemical cleaning products also have fragrances in them that should be avoided by people with asthma.

276.   If you have asthma, you are especially sensitive to things you breathe into your lungs. It is important to avoid whatever triggers your asthma. In some people, this will be cigarette smoke. For others, it is chemical fumes or other vapors that can irritate the lungs and bring on an attack.

277.   When it comes to asthma, many people have been known to abuse their inhalers without even realizing it. It is not a breath freshener, it is only to be used when you have a serious attack. Sometimes just simple calming breathing

techniques or stopping moving are all you need to stop an attack. Don't always resort to your inhaler as this can make your body stop reacting to it and make it useless.

278.   Every single week, get in the habit of washing your bed sheets. During the course of the day, dust mites will reside on your bed, which can incite symptoms of asthma when you sleep. Clean your sheets to eliminate this dust mites and create a hygienic area for resting.

279.   Attending asthma support group meetings, or even talking to a few chosen people with the condition, can do wonders for you. People who have experience with the same disease as you can often provide a number of suggestions or tricks that work in specific situations - all of which can make your battle with asthma a little earlier. Surround yourself with people who understand asthma and support your fight against it.

280.   Researchers have found that Vitamin C plays a large role in keeping airways functioning normally. Low levels of vitamin C can prevent symptoms associated with airway diseases, such as asthma. It can also help to control the progression and severity of the disease.

281.   You do not have to be physically inactive just because you have asthma. Unlike decades ago, when asthma treatments were few and far between, there are plenty of different asthma inhalers and medications that you can take prior to and after performing physical activities. Ask your doctor for the best treatment for your specific needs.

282.   A good tip that can help you if your child has asthma is to do everything you can to educate your child about asthma. Young children have no idea what asthma is or how it affects them, so it's your job to inform them and to help them work through it.

283.   Leukotriene inhibitors may be helpful to you if you suffer from asthma. As its name suggests, this inhibitor works by preventing the release and build-up of leukotriene. A leukotriene will cause inflammation in the respiratory system, causing an asthma attack. Using an inhibitor will counteract the negative effects of leukotriene, thereby decreasing the occurrence of asthma attacks.

284.   Stop what you are doing when you feel that an asthma attack is coming. This is especially true when you are driving or operating heavy

machinery. Explain to the people around you what is going on as they may become overly excited which in return can stress you out even more.

285.   If you feel that your asthma symptoms are getting worse, try drinking a cup of hot coffee. Not only will the warmth relieve some of your symptoms, the caffeine can open up your airways and reduce the urge to cough. If you don't like coffee, try tea, hot chocolate, or a chocolate bar.

286.   When you are packing for a vacation and you have asthma, be sure to pack an extra rescue inhaler. In case your inhaler gets lost, having a back up will ensure that you do not go without medications. Also, do not forget to bring any pills you take for your asthma.

287.   When dealing with hay fever or a cold, you will notice an increase in your asthma symptoms. Many of these illnesses will worsen your asthma symptoms bad enough to require more treatments than you typically need. Your doctor may need to add new treatments to your typical asthma regimen until you are well.

288.   Asthma can range from a small annoyance to an all-out, life-threatening condition. To help

prevent Asthma attacks, keep moderation in mind, especially when engaging in outdoor activities in hot weather. Hot and humid air can make breathing difficult for anyone, but for someone with Asthma, it can be deadly. If you have work to do outside, try and choose to do so early in the morning or late in the day and avoid the mid-day sun and heat.

289.   If you are an asthma patient, be sure that you are drinking water that has been filtered. Unfiltered water could possibly contain allergens which could cause a severe asthma attack or flare up your symptoms. If you can afford it, you may want to consider only drinking water that has come from a bottle.

290.   When you are traveling, be sure to carry your rescue inhaler with you at all times. When you travel, you sometimes strain your body a little more than you think, which can make you a bit more susceptible to having asthma attacks. Traveling can make asthma symptoms worse, and it is difficult, nearly impossible to control environmental triggers during travel.

291.   Avoid all the things that trigger your asthma. Cigarette smoke can be especially troublesome, but there are other things to avoid. Stay indoors

during times when there may be a nearby fire because the soot and ash will aggravate your lungs and stay away from strong vapors and chemical fumes.

292.   Stay inside whenever it is humid or during times of high pollen. Springtime is nice, but not if you can't breathe and that is the season that is likely to cause the most aggravation to your asthma condition. Invite friends over and find indoor activities that you can enjoy during these times, so that you don't feel deprived from not being able to go outside.

293.   A common trigger of asthma is tobacco smoke. Smoke is an irritant and aggravates asthma. If you have asthma you should stay away from smoke and make sure no one smokes around you, in your car or in your home. It is possible your asthma could be also be irritated by fumes, strong odors, changes in weather, or air pollution.

294.   A doctor will generally prescribe two different asthma inhalers. One of them will be a brown inhaler which should be taken regularly, and the other will be a blue inhaler for emergencies. You should always carry your blue inhaler with you in case you have an asthma

attack, and make sure to stay on top of refilling the prescription as needed. In the event of an asthma attack, if the blue inhaler is not helping, do not hesitate to call 911.

295.   If you find yourself without an inhaler when an asthma attack is coming on, try having a cold soda. The caffeine can actually open your airways and control the asthma. Preferably keep your inhaler on you at all times, but in case you find yourself without one, try drinking a caffeinated beverage.

296.   Finding out as much as you can about asthma is a good way to help you manage your asthma. The greater your knowledge base regarding asthma, the more involved you can be in determining treatment plans. Keep current with treatments and ensure you have the greatest possible care that you can have. Make sure to explore new and different options to keep the symptoms of your condition under control.

297.   Think about getting a flu shot. If you have asthma regularly, your lungs have more risks have getting infected. A flu shot should protect your lungs from common types of infections. If you have a child with asthma, you should

definitely get them a flu shot to prevent them from developing any severe lung infections.

298.   A good tip if you're struggling with asthma is to make sure you talk to your doctor so you can figure out the best treatment. Sometimes your asthma might be too much for an inhaler to handle. Talking to your doctor will help you get the appropriate treatment you need.

299.   If your children have asthma or hives, they might actually have certain food allergies. You should go to a doctor and do the necessary tests to find out if they are allergic to something and then, make sure they stay away from that particular food, if they turn out to be allergic.

300.   It is important that you do not get too stressed out if you suffer from asthma. Stress and panic are all major causes of asthma attacks. Also, try not lose your temper either. Getting angry can cause your breathing to become labored, which in turn, can trigger asthma attacks.

301.   Medications can be taken on a regular basis to control inflammation in your airways. Inhaled corticosteroids such as cromolyn and leukotriene modifiers are some such medications. Consult

with your doctor about which one is the best for you. You may need to try several of them.

302.   When dealing with asthma, you should limit your contact with animals. Many people who have asthma also have an allergy to pets. Even if you do not have an allergy to pets, pets can carry trigger substances, such as dirt, in their fur. These substances could cause an attack without you being allergic to pets.

303.   Having the proper medications and treatments for your asthma is very important. If you need to use your inhaler more than once a day, or are awakened by symptoms more than twice a week, it may be time to switch to a more controlling medicine that can prevent your symptoms.

304.   Be aware of how your diet affects your asthma. Often specific foods like peanut butter contain allergens for anyone suffering from asthma. If you have certain food-based triggers, manage your diet to avoid those ingredients and lessen your asthma symptoms and attacks. If you try a new food, monitor your symptoms to ensure it does not cause increased asthma problems.

305.   Engage your support network to help you manage your asthma. Talk to your friends and family about items that trigger attacks and enroll them in helping you make environmental or lifestyle changes to help you manage your asthma. The more knowledgeable your network is about your condition, the more easily they can support you.

306.   Be your child's asthma advocate, especially at school. Many schools have policies in place that prohibit children from carrying medications on them. This is not acceptable when it comes to an emergency rescue inhaler. Find out what steps you need to take to make sure that your child has access to their medication as needed.

307.   Don't smoke. People know that smoking is dangerous, but it is even more dangerous to those with asthma. An asthmatic's lungs are more vulnerable than those of a healthy individual, which makes it especially important to abstain from smoking and avoid secondhand smoke.

308.   Asthma sufferers need to stay inside as much as they can when the air's pollen content is high. While asthma isn't an allergy, many allergy irritants can affect it. Asthma suffers can now

minimize exposure to outdoor pollutants and irritants by checking online for current air quality in their areas.

309. If you have asthma, it is important to avoid allergens. These irritants can trigger an attack and cause coughing, wheezing and shortness of breath. Things you should stay away from are tobacco smoke, pollen, dust, mold and pet dander. Some people are also sensitive to cold air or overexerting themselves.

310. It is important to stay indoors during certain seasons when you have asthma. Some times of the year when the air is especially humid, spending too much time outdoors can make it difficult for you to breathe. Other times, the pollen count gets very high and can trigger an asthma attack.

311. Try to identify situations that trigger your asthma attacks and avoid them. Some people tend to have noticeable triggers such as too much excitement, allergic reactions that cause breathing problems or a change of environment. If you can identify some of your triggers, try to avoid them to manage your asthma.

312.   Exercise is one of the most important things that you can do if you have asthma. Go to the gym at least three times per week and give your muscles a workout. This will allow your body the time to adjust and build its capacity to reduce your asthma symptoms.

313.   One important thing to remember when it comes to asthma is that different triggers are more or less severe for different people. While tobacco smoke may trigger a severe outbreak in one, it causes nothing in the other. As such work with your doctor to determine which triggers you need to avoid.

314.   Exercise moderately when you have asthma. Very strenuous exercise and the increased rate of breathing required can cause problems and trigger an asthma attack. Control your breathing by taking up light to moderate exercise. Yoga is especially helpful in this regard. Swimming may also help with breath control while providing good exercise.